got fibroids?®

got fibroids?®

The Fibroid Elimination Bible

The comprehensive all-natural system of eliminating women's reproductive disorders.

electric pHood™

2020

Cover Design By Heka Multimedia

Layout By Emykhet Akhu Kinshaye

Printed and bound in the United States of America

First Edition

ISBN 978-0-578-65598-7 (pbk.)

TABLE OF CONTENTS

PREFACE

A message from the electric Docs™, Dr. Amsu Anpu & Dr. Amun Neb:

We hope that you are as enthusiastic about starting this life-changing journey that you are about to embark upon, as we are for you. If you are committed to following this fibroid elimination program, willing to try new things, and most importantly, willing to let go of old habits, we can promise you that you won't walk away dissatisfied.

If you are asking yourself the **question** "why is my body failing me?" we are here to assure you that, on the contrary, your body is behaving well within its naturally programmed bounds, and it is only trying to survive the perpetual onslaught of toxins (poisons) that you have subjected it to, through your modern lifestyle – toxic foods, toxic drinks, toxic air, and toxic exercises. These toxins are the root cause to your body's imbalance and adverse reaction: INFLAMMATION.

Our Fibroid Elimination Bible is exactly what you need, whether you are suffering from uterine fibroids, cysts or any other reproductive growth disorder. The basic premise of The Fibroid Elimination Bible is that by creating the right conditions, your body will begin to naturally heal itself. How? Through removing the major toxins, and feeding your body essential, nutritionally-beneficial foods and natural, mineral rich supplements.

To begin you must first admit and affirm, with powerful desire, to change your old/bad habits which are responsible for your body being in its undesirable and dysfunctional state. The elimination program begins with the tackling and extraction of toxins from your body, which will be a great benefit. The program then focuses on replenishing your body with the correct nutrients and minerals to regenerate red blood cells, and to repair damaged organs and muscle tissue.

Remember that, throughout your experience, we are addressing the root causes of the toxins that cause imbalance and, therefore, inhibit you from having a healthy body. Rest assured that the Team will be there to guide you through this journey every step of the way.

Thousands of women have successfully eliminated their fibroids and cysts using our Fibroid Elimination Bible program, and are now enjoying healthy reproductive lives. We hope that after this experience, we can add your name to this list.

Here's to your optimum health.

Electric Health is comprised of top Endocrinologists, Naturopaths, Herbalists, Nutritionists and Dietitians. We are NOT MD's. This means we are neither pressured nor do we conform to the allopathic and pharmacological ideologies that control the conventional healthcare and medical industries. Our natural approach to disease reversal means that we focus our energies on finding the most effective, natural remedies to the many diseases that we overcome, and are not bound by local or federal regulations that would force us to compromise and conform to their allopathic standards. One of the unique principals that our practitioners exercise is the continued education of our expert consultants, who actually study the thousands of white papers released by the world's leading research scientists in the medical and healing fields, so we are fully aware of all the latest medical advancements and discoveries that are most often contrary to the practices of conventional MDs. We then incorporate the best of this wide body of information into our practices to produce the best healing remedies and protocols. This education is then passed on to you, our client, so that you know exactly what is going on in your body, and thus can make an educated decision about how best to proceed in your related healing.

INTRODUCTION

You are reading this instructional manual because you are either considering an alternative to the popularized procedures that have been strongly advocated, if not dictated, by the well-established medical institutions, or you have made an actual decision to forgo the advice and recommendation of your gynecologist, and choose the natural and best remedy to eliminate your fibroids.

The Statistics

80% of all women in the United States will suffer from fibroids. Only a small percentage suffer from the symptoms, so the condition often remains unreported to physicians and gynecologists until the fibroids mature into large tumors. At this point most gynecologists have only one procedure in mind to treat the affliction: **Hysterectomy**.

Hysterectomy

Hysterectomy is the surgical removal of the uterus. It may also involve removal of the cervix, ovaries, fallopian tubes and other surrounding structures. Usually performed by a gynecologist, hysterectomy may be **total** (removing the body, fundus, and cervix of the uterus; often called "complete") or **partial** (removal of the uterine body while leaving the cervix intact; also called "supracervical"). It is the most commonly performed gynecological surgical procedure. Removal of the uterus renders the patient unable to bear children (as does removal of ovaries and fallopian tubes) and has surgical risks as well as long-term negative effects.

The United States performs more hysterectomies than any other country in the world. There are over 600,000 hysterectomies performed in the United States each year, over 300,000 of which are due to uterine fibroids. An overwhelming 78% of all the U.S. hysterectomies are performed on African-American women, which means that there are 468,000 African-American hysterectomies per year, and that over 234,000 of them are due to fibroids. Such rates being highest in the industrialized world has led to the major controversy that hysterectomies are being largely performed for unwarranted and unnecessary reasons.

Over $5Billion is spent each year on just the hysterectomy procedure. An additional $5Billion is spent on post-hysterectomy treatment and medication, such as hormone therapy. According to a report published by Obstetrics & Gynecology, 75% of hysterectomies do not follow the American College of Obstetricians and Gynecologists (ACOG) Guidelines for offering alternative procedural treatment options. So, basically, there are other alternatives to a hysterectomy that are neither disclosed nor discussed by gynecologists to their fibroid-suffering patients.

Other Surgical/Non-Surgical Procedures

Oophorectomy

An oophorectomy (removal of ovaries) is frequently done together with hysterectomy to decrease the risk of ovarian cancer. However, recent studies have shown that prophylactic oophorectomy without an urgent medical indication decreases a woman's long-term survival rates substantially and has other serious adverse effects. This effect is not limited to pre-menopausal women; even women who have already entered menopause were shown to have experienced a decrease in long-term survivability post-oophorectomy.

Myomectomy/Fibroidectomy

A myomectomy is the surgical removal of just the fibroids. This alternative procedure is dependent upon the size and location of the fibroids. It can be performed hysteroscopically, laparoscopically, or through abdominal surgery. Although gynecologists do receive training for these three procedures, not all are skilled enough to perform them. The result, a gynecologist's recommendations for treatment may rest solely, or at least partially, on his actual skill and, therefore, his comfort level for performing a procedure, than it has to do with what is best for the patient's medical condition. As a result, the cost of a myomectomy is considerably higher than a hysterectomy, with the lowest national price at approximately $10,000 for the procedure.

Uterine Artery Embolization

Uterine Artery Embolization (UAE also known as UFE for Uterine Fibroid Embolization): a procedure performed exclusively by an interventional radiologist, which involves the placement of minute polyvinyl (plastic) particles into the uterine artery that feeds the fibroid tumors. It's a relatively simple and non-invasive procedure that severs the blood supply feeding the uterine fibroids. Without the blood supply, the fibroids die and then shrink. UAE has been around for over 20 years, and is used, primarily, for stopping hemorrhaging after childbirth or surgery. It is only within the past decade that gynecologists have started collaborating with interventional radiologists to introduce this procedure as a standard non-surgical option for the treatment of uterine fibroids. Despite the fact that gynecologists do not perform the procedure, and that by referring women for this procedure in lieu of a hysterectomy, and that gynecologists will lose the surgical fees involved, some gynecologists have somehow worked their respective fees into the procedure and this technique is being widely popularized as the best and only solution to fibroids, whilst demonizing its surgical counterparts.

Myolysis

Myolysis (myoma coagulation) procedure also cuts off the blood supply to the fibroids, and causes them to wither and die. Patients begin with several months of treatment with a gonadotropin releasing hormone (GnRH) agonist such as Lupron, a drug given by injection, to shrink the fibroids as much as possible, and then laparoscopic surgery is performed. Through laparoscopy, a laser pierces the fibroids, and electrical charges are sent to the fibroids to destroy the blood vessels.

Out of the Proverbial Frying Pan

It is eHealth's stance that UAE is being falsely perpetrated as the savior for women with fibroids. There are significant risk factors associated with UAE that, unfortunately, have not been publicized. These risks include:

- Death from Embolism
- Death from Septicemia

- The presence of pus-forming or other pathogenic organisms, or their toxins, in the blood or tissues resulting in multiple organ failure

- Infection from tissue death of fibroids leading to endometritis
- Misembolization from microspheres
- Particles flowing or drifting into other tissues
- Ovarian damage
- Embolic material migrating to the ovaries
- Loss of ovarian function; infertility; loss of orgasm
- Post-Embolization Syndrome
- Acute / chronic pain; up to 102 degree temperatures, nausea, vomiting

Uterine Artery Embolization Procedure

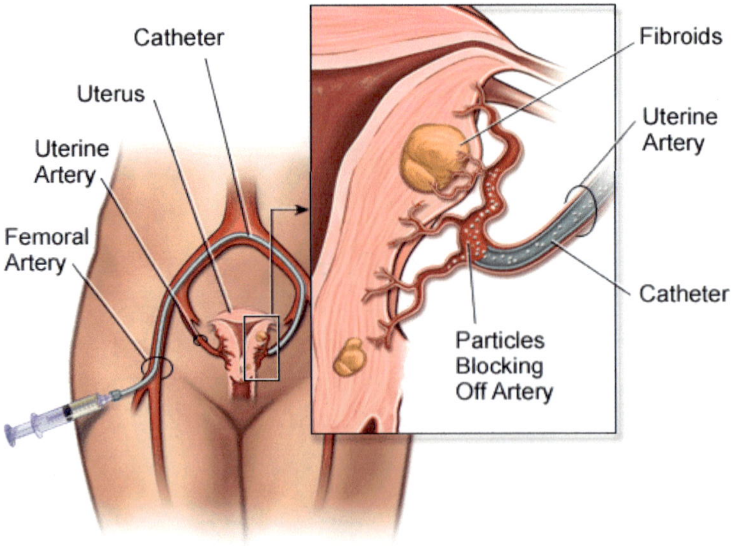

ARE YOU READY TO START ELIMINATING YOUR FIBROIDS?

CHAPTER 1

Women's Reproductive Disorders

JUST WHAT ARE FIBROIDS?

Common name: Uterine Fibroids

Medical name: Uterine Leiomyomata

Uterine fibroids are tumors or lumps made of muscle cells and other tissue that grow within the walls of the uterus. Fibroids may grow as a single tumor or in clusters. A single fibroid can be less than one inch in size or can grow to eight inches across or more. A bunch or cluster of fibroids can all vary in size. Uterine fibroids are the most common, non-cancerous tumors in women of childbearing age.

Most fibroids grow within the walls of the uterus. Healthcare providers classify fibroids into three groups based on where they grow:

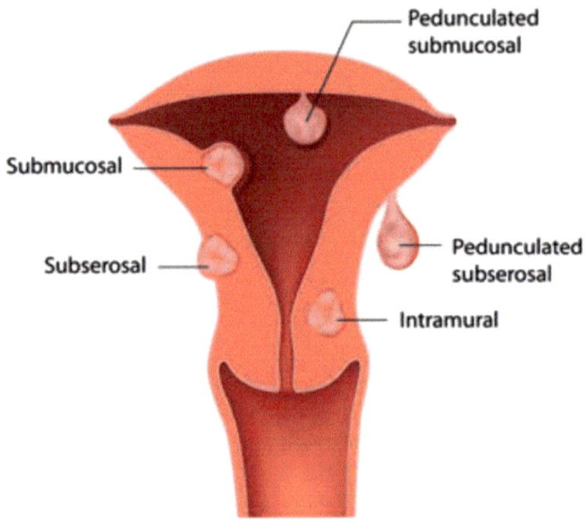

a) Submucosal fibroids grow just underneath the uterine lining.

b) Intramural fibroids grow in between the muscles of the uterus.

c) Subserosal fibroids grow on the outside of the uterus.

WHAT ABOUT CYSTS?

Cysts differ from fibroids, in that they are fluid filled sacs which can develop anywhere on the body. There are several different types of ovarian cysts:

Functional Cysts (so-called*) - These cysts form during the "normal" menstrual cycle. A sac containing eggs forms and usually breaks open to release the egg and the sac dissolves. Sometimes, the sac doesn't break open and continues to grow. This is called a follicular cyst. It usually disappears in 30 to 90 days. Another type which have been erroneously labeled as "functional" cysts, are called Corpus Luteum Cysts which occur when the corpus luteum sac doesn't dissolve right away. This usually disappears on its own in a few weeks.

* It is eHealth's position that the menstrual cycle, and in particular, the luteinizing phase, is an unnatural phenomenon but has become the norm amid the "nitrogen fixation cycle", which will be discussed later in this publication.

Endometriomas - This type of cyst can develop in women who have endometriosis. Tissue from the lining of the uterus grows outside the uterus and if it attaches to the ovary it can cause a cyst.

Cystadenomas - This type of cyst forms from the outer cells of the ovary.

Dermoid Cysts (Teratomas) - Cells in the ovary which develop hair, teeth or other tissue during pregnancy can become part of an ovarian cyst. When this happens, it is called a dermoid cyst.

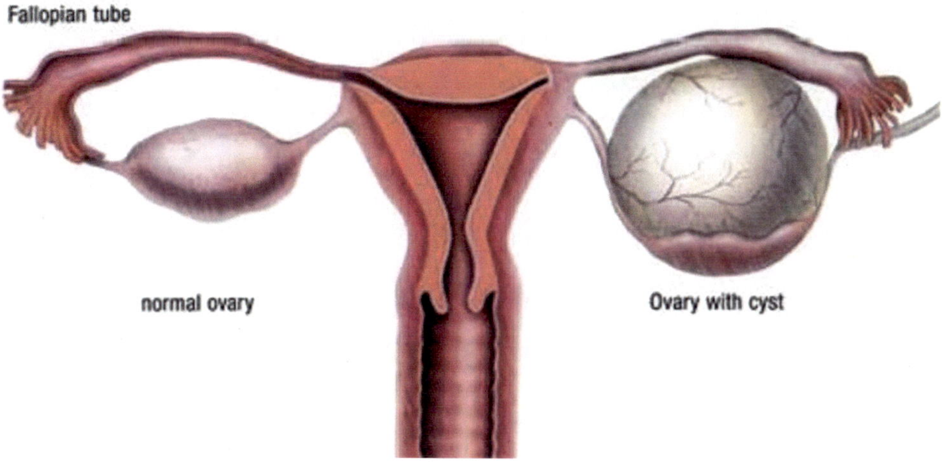

ENDOMETRIOSIS

Endometriosis is a chronic inflammatory disease in which the lining of the uterus (endometrium) is found or grows outside of the uterus. It is the most common cause of pelvic pain and occurs in 30 – 40% of women with infertility. Endometriosis is the third leading cause of gynecological hospitalization in the US. It is commonly characterized by:

- pathological lesions or nodules - solid, damaged raised skin
- implants - endometrial tissue found in ectopic locations
- adhesions - scar tissue
- endometritis - inflammation of the inner lining of the uterus (endometrium)
- pyometra - an intrauterine infection and collection of pus-filled material due to the inability of the cervix to adequately drain uterine contents
- glandular cystic hyperplasia - a condition, caused by too much estrogen (or too little progesterone) in which the endometrium is abnormally thick. It is not cancer but, in some cases, it can lead to cancer of the uterus. There are four types of endometrial hyperplasia:
    - simple endometrial hyperplasia
    - complex endometrial hyperplasia
    - simple atypical endometrial hyperplasia
    - complex atypical endometrial hyperplasia

ENDOMETRIOSIS

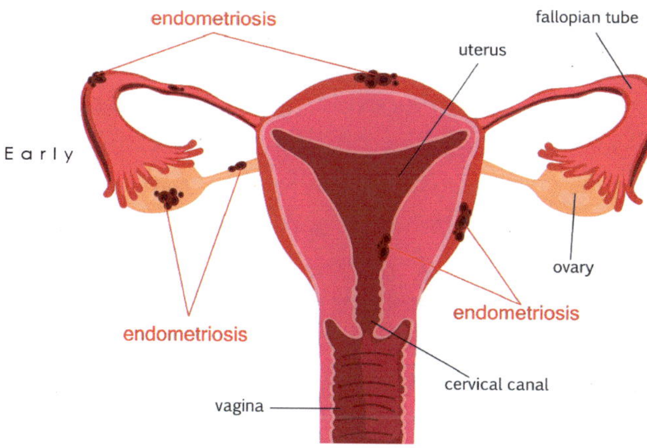

Early pregnancy loss, a common but severe occurrence among sufferers, may be caused by mechanical obstruction of implantation or distortion of the cervix or endometrium. There are 4 stages of endometriosis:

- Stage 1: Minimal implanted tissue deposits and lesions with no significant adhesions
- Stage 2: Mild - superficial implants and lesions measuring up to 5cm without significant adhesions
- Stage 3: Moderate - multiple deep implants, small cysts on one or both ovaries, and the presence of flimsy adhesions
- Stage 4: Severe - multiple deep implants, large cysts on one or both ovaries, and thick adhesions.

SYMPTOMS OF ENDOMETRIOSIS

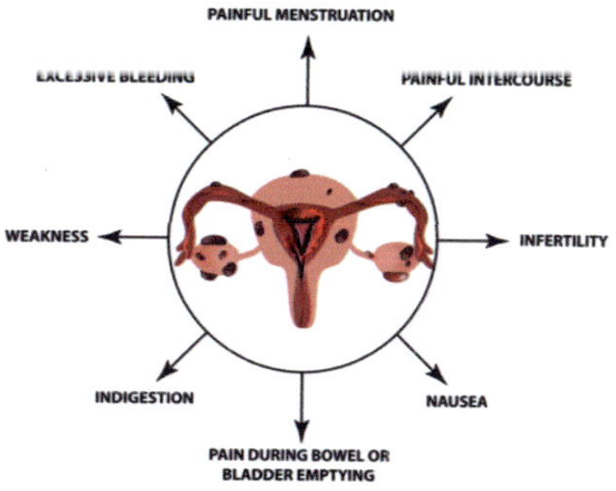

Each Stage also signifies an increasing level of pain ranging from discomfort to extremely debilitating. Endometriosis tissue can spread throughout the body. It has been found in every organ and anatomical structure in the body except the spleen. The lower abdominal cavity (pelvic cavity), however, is the most common general area where endometriosis occurs, and the most common cites include the peritoneum (lining of the pelvic area), the rectouterine pouch (also called the Pouch of Douglas or cul-de-sac), the rectovaginal septum, the uterosacral ligaments, the ovaries, the fallopian tubes, all over the outside of the uterus, including underneath it and behind it, the appendix, bowel, bladder, and the rectum. Although exceedingly rare, endometriosis can invade other vital organs and structures such as the kidneys, the eyes, liver, pancreas, bone, heart, skin, nasal cavity, and even the brain. When endometriosis tissue invades the brain, it is called cerebral endometriosis.

Those Darn Headaches

Endometriosis has been closely linked with migraine headaches. Although migraine and endometriosis blatantly affect different parts of the body, they share similar clinical and epidemiological features, most of which can be accounted for by the influence of female sex hormones, in particular estrogen, on both disorders.

Early menarche (the first occurrence of menstruation) seems to be a risk factor for both headache and endometriosis. For migraines, it is curious that the age of menarche seems to influence the prevalence of headache, not only among adolescents but throughout life of those affected. Many aspects linking psychological factors related to early physical maturation, to physiological factors related to higher estrogen levels (or to increased estrogen sensitivity), have been raised to explain why headache is more prevalent in females with early menarche.

Adenomyosis

Adenomyosis is a specific form of endometriosis where the lining grows deep into the muscle wall of the uterus and thickens it. Unlike endometriosis, adenomyosis doesn't go past the uterus itself. It's sometimes called internal endometriosis.

POLYCYSTIC OVARY SYNDROME

Polycystic ovary syndrome (PCOS) is a highly prevalent, complex reproductive endocrine disorder that is fundamentally characterized by polycystic ovaries, chronic anovulation and hyperandrogenism leading to symptoms of irregular menstrual cycles, hirsutism, acne and infertility. Different PCOS experts adjudicate the effects of PCOS based upon their field of expertise - some specialize in metabolism, blood sugar levels and insulin, seeing PCOS primarily as a risk for diabetes and obesity. Others that are skin experts see the skin oiliness, acne, and unwanted facial and body hair as typical of PCOS. As an endocrinologist, specializing in hormones and glands, I've taken a giant step back to look at the entire picture that encompasses all the changes that characterize the experiences of PCOS in entire populations of women.

Hormonal interactions in PCOS

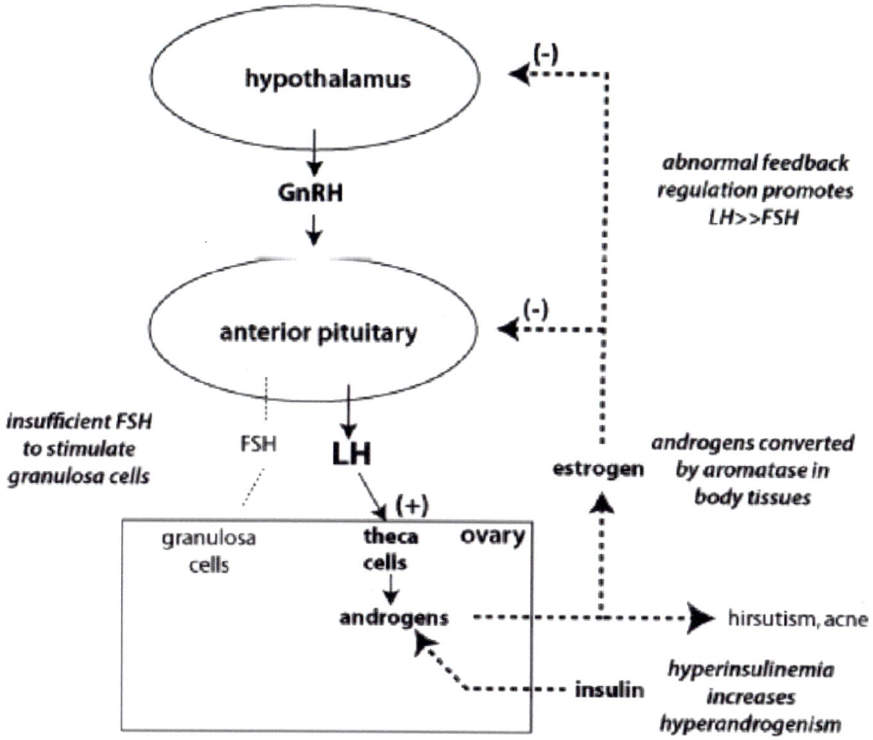

It is the position of the electric Docs that the underlying mechanism of PCOS falls on estrogen dominance and the eventual overproduction of another hormone called gonadotropin releasing hormone (GnRH). Normally, the hypothalamus, a regulatory center in the brain, monitors the hormone output of the ovaries and synchronizes the normal menstrual cycle. When monthly bleeding ends, the hypothalamus secretes gonadotropin-releasing hormone (GnRH), which stimulates the ***pituitary gland*** (a small hormone producing gland at the base of the brain) to release follicle stimulating hormone (FSH) and luteinizing hormone (LH). Unopposed estrogen interferes with operation of the hypothalamus, causing GnRH to be released too rapidly, that is, it is not properly regulated, and is released in a frequency much higher than normal ***pulses***. This, in turn, leads to rapid pulses of LH from the pituitary gland. This endocrine disruption of the pituitary gland causes a simultaneous inhibition of FSH. The release of too much LH and too little FSH may (and often does) stimulate higher levels of androgens (including testosterone) to be produced in the ovaries which interfere with ovulation and the menstrual cycle. These androgens are then aromatized into more estrogen, which causes greater dysfunction of the hypothalamus gland and pituitary gland, releasing even more GnRH and more LH, respectively, and the cycle continues. We call this ***abnormal feedback regulation***.

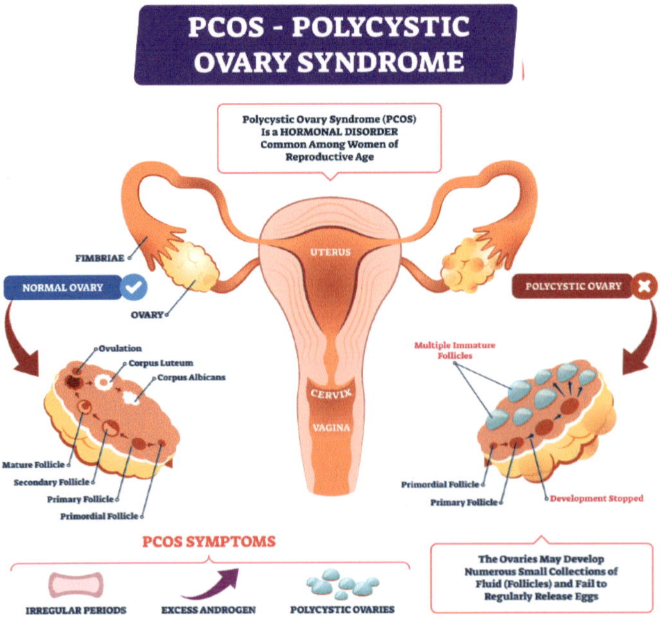

THOSE UNPLEASANT SYMPTOMS!!!

Female reproductive disorders share common symptoms. They will vary according to the individual's root causes and by differing biological dispositions, but below is a list of the main culprits among which you are experiencing:

- Achiness in lower back
- Problems urinating
- Pelvic pain
- Pain during sex
- Weight gain (Obesity)
- Abnormal bleeding or more pain during your menstrual cycle than normal
- Nausea and/or vomiting
- Tenderness in your breasts
- Anemia
- Miscarriage
- Infertility

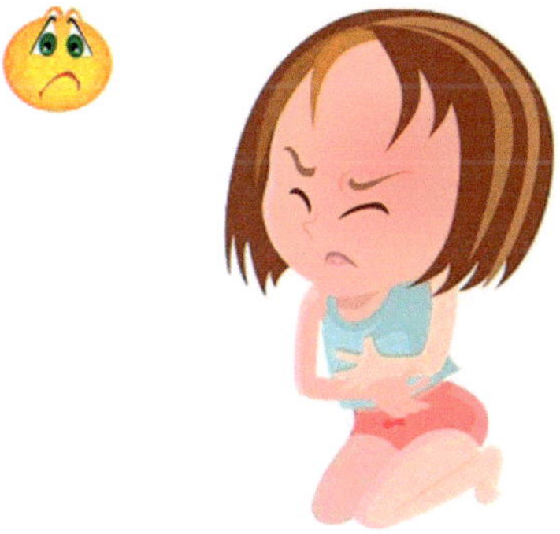

Upon completion of our HerElimination™ program you will be free of all associated fibroids/cysts/endometriosis/PCOS symptoms.

MORE PAIN THAN PLEASURE

Keep That Thing Away from Me

Fibroids are the result, inter alia, of an endocrinal dysfunction - as will be revealed shortly – which means there are persistent hormonal imbalances. **"Hormones"** is just a fancy word for biological chemicals that are produced by various glands within the body. The master glands are found in the brain, and the respondent/receptor glands are distributed within the internal boundaries of the torso. These chemicals absolutely control and influence your moods and behavior, including your responses or reactions to any given external phenomena.

Sexual activity, being of the most overtly hormone-influenced behaviors, is affected immensely by fibroids. The sufferer may not only experience increasingly painful sexual intercourse, but may also exhibit a rapidly diminishing libido, as the **limbic system** is often the first bio-chemical mechanism to fall prey prior to, and during the onset of the growths. The **limbic system** is the area of the brain that sees most of your sexual chemical activity. It is the seat of your emotions, drives, impulses and desires – especially sexual ones. It is where you instinctively fall in and out of love, and in and out of lust. The limbic system's job is quite simply to keep you alive and reproducing, and it performs this fundamental job by mandating you to avoid pain, and to replicate what is pleasurable. The precursor and, or aftermath to fibroids is the disruption in production of the sexual and emotional chemicals manufactured in the limbic system, namely dopamine, **oxytocin** and **vasopressin**.

Dopamine is a natural chemical and neurotransmitter that helps you to maintain an optimum level of brain stimulation. It stimulates 'desire and reward' by triggering an intense rush of pleasure. It has the same effect on the brain as taking cocaine, hence its derived term "dope". Outside the nervous system, dopamine functions in several parts of the body as a local chemical messenger. In the blood vessels, it inhibits norepinephrine – a neurotransmitter that causes tension of vascular smooth muscles (amongst other functions) - release and acts as a vasodilator; in the kidneys, it increases sodium excretion and urine output; in the pancreas, it reduces insulin production; in the digestive system, it reduces gastrointestinal motility and protects intestinal mucosa; and it maintains immune system purity, by reducing the activity of lymphocytes (white blood cells).

Oxytocin plays an important role in the neuroanatomy of intimacy, specifically in sexual reproduction. It has an important and immediate role in various behaviors, including sexual arousal, orgasm, social recognition, pair bonding, anxiety, and maternal response. Oxytocin evokes feelings of contentment, reductions in anxiety, and feelings of calmness and security around one's partner. Oxytocin is important for the inhibition of the brain regions associated with behavioral control, fear, and anxiety. It also functions to protect against stress.

Vasopressin has a variety of neurological effects on the brain, having been found to influence pair-bonding, social behavior, sexual motivation, sexual satisfaction, aggression, affection, and maternal responses to stress. Its primary functions, though, are to retain water in the body and to constrict blood vessels. Vasopressin regulates the body's retention of water by acting to increase water reabsorption in the collecting ducts of the kidneys.

VAGINAL YEAST INFECTIONS

A vaginal yeast infection is a type of vaginitis — inflammation of the vagina characterized by vaginal irritation, intense itchiness and vaginal discharge. A vaginal yeast infection affects your vagina and the tissues at the opening to your vagina (vulva). It is caused by the fungal organism Candida Albicans Candida Albicans feed on Vitamin B7, or hybridized/synthetic glucose. They need excess estrogen to survive. Estrogen influences vaginal glucose/glycogen levels.

Vaginal yeast infection — also called vaginal candidiasis — is very common. As many as 3 out of 4 women experience a yeast infection at some point in their lifetimes. Many women experience two or more yeast infections.

A vaginal yeast infection isn't considered a sexually transmitted infection, although the fungus that causes the condition can be spread through oral-genital contact.

Yeast infection symptoms can range from mild to moderate and include:

- Itching and irritation in the vagina and at the entrance to the vagina (vulva)
- A burning sensation, especially during intercourse or while urinating
- Redness and swelling of the vulva
- Vaginal pain and soreness
- Thick, white, odor-free vaginal discharge with a cottage cheese appearance

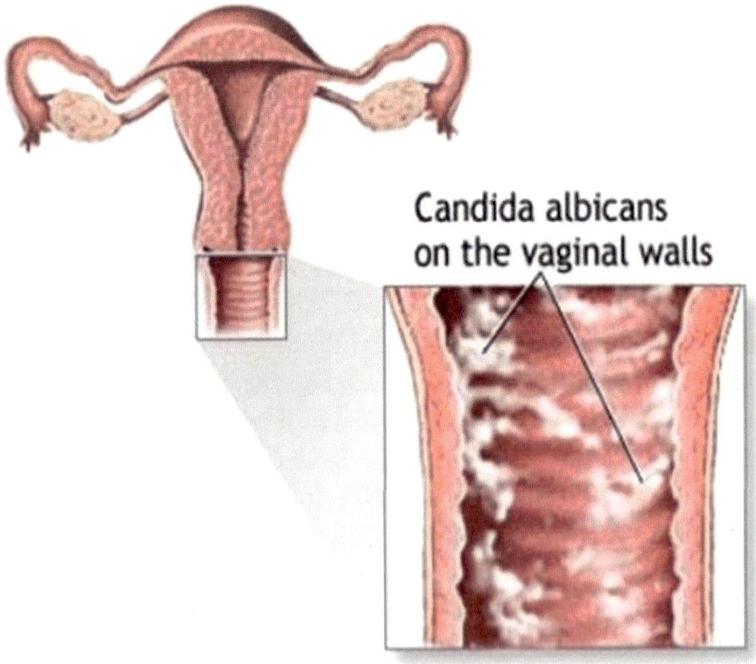

CHAPTER 2

The Common Cause

Despite the concerted effort to conceal the root cause of these reproductive disorders, by the American Medical Association (AMA), the World Health Organization (WHO), and various other western medical institutions, electric Health has not only identified the culprit, but is making every effort to totally eradicate this fiendish chemical out of the human biology.

What is it then?

It is none other than **ESTROGEN...** Yes estrogen...you know the "hormone" that, supposedly, differentiates women from men. The fact is estrogen is NOT a natural hormone. In fact, estrogen is a known and documented carcinogen...yes, it's cancerous. Numerous white papers from multiple scientific and medical research institutions have confirmed and reaffirmed it. But this information is not being disseminated to the general, "consumer" public.

There are three major types of estrogens that occur endogenously in women:

- Estrone (E1)
- Estradiol (E2)
- Estriol (E3)

They are steroidal, and as such readily diffuse across the cell membrane. Once inside the cell, they bind to and activate estrogen receptors which in turn modulate, or mutate the expression of many genes (and therefore the cells).

The general consensus amongst the western medical community is to promote that there is "NO KNOWN CAUSE FOR FIBROIDS" whilst recommending and prescribing estrogen pills to childbearing women of all ages to "regulate" heavy menstrual cycles, and ease the symptoms of ovarian cysts.

It is eHealth's stance that the end game is to increase the count of uterine fibroids and cysts to generate the perpetual economy and revenue stream that comes as a result of the wide scale hysterectomy and myomectomy operations, and the other alternate procedures, such as Uterine Fibroid Embolization/

Uterine Artery Embolization (UFE/UAE).

Estrogen is known to cause or advance the following diseases and conditions:

Cancers: (see https://ehoonline.biomedcentral.com/articles/10.1186/s40164-018-0116-7)	
Breast	(see http://www.ncbi.nlm.nih.gov/pubmed/17113977)
Ovarian	(see https://www.ncbi.nlm.nih.gov/pmc/articles/PMC4228918/)
Endometrial	(see https://www.acog.org/Patients/FAQs/Endometrial-Cancer?IsMobileSet=false)
Lung	(see https://www.ncbi.nlm.nih.gov/pmc/articles/PMC2928145/)

Diseases & Conditions	
Lupus	(see https://lupusnewstoday.com/2016/01/21/the-immune-system-is-a-natural-target-for-estrogen-action-opposing-effects-of-estrogen-in-two-prototypical-autoimmune-diseases/)
Thyroiditis	(see https://www.ncbi.nlm.nih.gov/pmc/articles/PMC3113168/)
Cervical Dysplasia	(see https://erc.bioscientifica.com/view/journals/erc/24/4/R99.xml)
Fibrocystic breasts	(see https://www.ncbi.nlm.nih.gov/pubmed/3511705)
Gallbladder Disease	(see https://www.ncbi.nlm.nih.gov/pubmed/3732993)
Hair Loss	(see https://www.huffpost.com/entry/women-hair-loss_b_2597382)
Hypoglycemia	(see https://www.ncbi.nlm.nih.gov/pubmed/29224103)
Polycystic Ovaries	(see https://www.verywellhealth.com/estrogen-dominance-in-pcos-2616555)

Prostate Cancer (men only) (see https://www.ncbi.nlm.nih.gov/pmc/articles/PMC3134227/)

Water Retention (Bloating) (see https://www.ncbi.nlm.nih.gov/pmc/articles/PMC2849969/#S8title)

Estrogen decides body fat distribution, and, in women, fat is stored on the hips, buttocks, abdomen and thighs. Fat cells (white adipose tissue) manufacture and store estrogen, so the elimination of fat will also increase/expedite the desired elimination of your fibroids. Remember, this is always the same for cysts and yeast infections.

Exogenous estrogen is introduced into the body via food ingestion, and through the polluted atmosphere, in the form of ***Aromatas***

Aromatase:

- is also called estrogen synthetase or estrogen synthase
- is an enzyme responsible for a key step in the biosynthesis of estrogens
- is responsible for the aromatization of androgens into estrogens
- transforms androstenedione to estrone and testosterone to estradiol (E2)
- Is found in tissue of endometriosis, uterine fibroids, breast cancer, and endometrial cancer
- Inhibits the spin of the mitochondria = diminished cellular health/energy

IT IS THIS ENZYME THAT MUST BE ELIMINATED FROM YOUR DIET!!!

CHAPTER 3

Aromatase Based Foods

This is the short list of foods that you MUST eliminate immediately and permanently from your diet to exterminate your fibroids:

- Tofu
- Soybeans
- Soy Protein Isolate
- Sunflower
- Soybean Oil
- Safflower Oil
- Corn Oil
- Alcohol
- Cheese o Milk
- Legumes
- ALL MEATS

AROMATASE INHIBITORS

This is the first/short list of organic/wild foods that you MUST incorporate indefinitely into your diet to exterminate your fibroids:

- Blueberries
- Celery
- Black Cherries
- Purple Grapes (purple grape juice)
- Horseradish
- Kale (Dinosaur Kale is best) – Eat ONLY after Phase 3
- Roma and/or Grape Tomatoes (raw & unrefrigerated)
- Broccoli – Eat ONLY after Phase 3
- Green and especially Red Cabbage
- Cauliflower

CHAPTER 4

You Are What You Eat... Literally

Those old adages we hear so often throughout our lives, that we take for granted , or brush off as old wives tales and figures of speech, could not be truer.

We have all been victims of a "modern scientific bamboozle". We were all (and still are) taught that blood is created (hematopoiesis) in the bone marrow. This erroneous theory has been perpetuated, unchallenged, in the west for but a few centuries. Prior to this scientific farce, medicine and anatomy were advanced practices of the east, where the simple anatomic structure, as the basis for all animals, was well documented.

The animal's body, including humans, is comprised of three elements:

- Body cells
- A digestive system (Intestines)
- Blood cells

Body cells are made up of red blood cells. Red blood cells are produced in the mucous membrane of the intestines. Red blood corpuscle mother cells, which produce red blood cells, can only be found in the mucous membranes (intestinal villus structure) of the intestines. They are not found in the bone marrow, or anywhere else in the body. The intestines are the digestive system of the body. The digestive function of the digestive system is really the blood-making function of the body. Food is digested by the action of digestive enzymes, the churning action by the vermicular movement of the intestines, and bacteria in the intestines. The food, by the time it gets to the small intestines, is dissolved to a moneran (living matter) state. The food, in its moneran state, sticks to the mucous membranes of the intestinal walls. The intestinal villus structure takes the food moneran into its cells (chorioepithelial cells). The cells, in turn, digest the moneran, and they produce red corpuscle mother cells from it. The mother cells then produce red blood cells within themselves and attach themselves to the capillaries, which run through the center of the villus structure, and send them into the bloodstream. This is literally how the food you eat is transformed into your blood cells. Your blood cells then, amongst other functions, produce the cells that make up your body cells, tissues and organs.

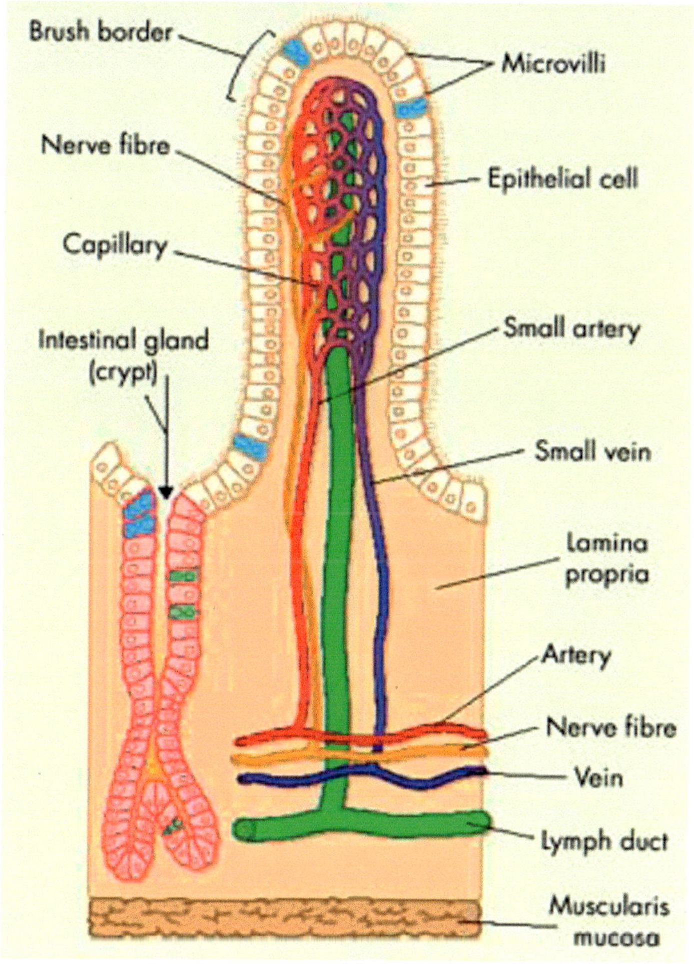
Brush border
Microvilli
Nerve fibre
Epithelial cell
Capillary
Small artery
Intestinal gland
(crypt)
Small vein
Lamina
propria
Artery
Nerve fibre
Vein
Lymph duct
Muscularis
mucosa

CHAPTER 5

Fat & Fibroids

It is no coincidence that the ratios shown in the comparison between races are directly proportionate with overweight and obesity statistics as those with fibroids and hysterectomies. According to the CDC 4 out of 5 African-American women are overweight or obese, and are 80% more likely to be obese than Non-Hispanic Whites. These same numbers are almost identically reflected in hysterectomy cases due to fibroids. The fact is the relationship shared between fat and fibroids is a direct and everlasting one. You are considered overweight if you have a Body Mass Index (BMI) of 25 or greater, and obese if your BMI is 30 or greater.

What is fat?

The term "fat" is an extremely vague one, as it can be attributed to several substances, such as fatty acids, oils, or lipids, that can either be loosely or closely related; so for clarity we will use the specific scientific term **white adipose tissue** when referring to unwanted body fat.

On the subject of white adipose tissue, the scientific and medical institutions, and their respective communities, are in much disarray as to its functional/ dysfunctional nature and behavior. This is mainly due to the fact that the term "adipose tissue" which also includes **brown adipose tissue** – the natural and functional adipose tissue - is often used synonymously with white adipose tissue.

White adipose tissue is not a natural component of our bodies. It is the result of the ingestion of non-digestible substances, i.e. substances that are not properly processed by the digestive system and are instead deposited at low electrically-charged sites around the body. These low electrically-charged sites are known as our intrinsic **weak spots**, and become, as a result, target areas and havens for parasites (viruses, fungi and bacteria).

Medical Complications of Obesity

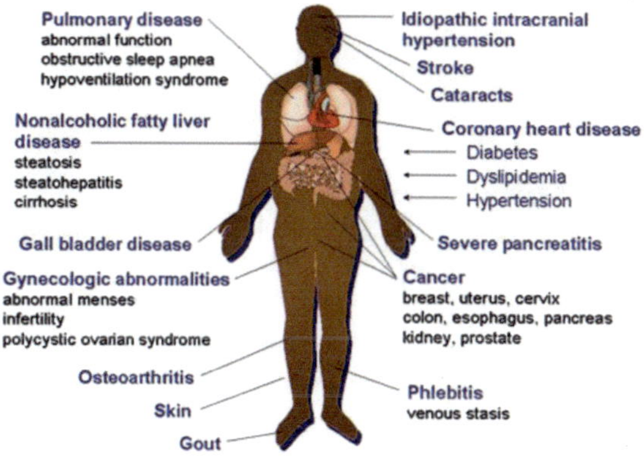

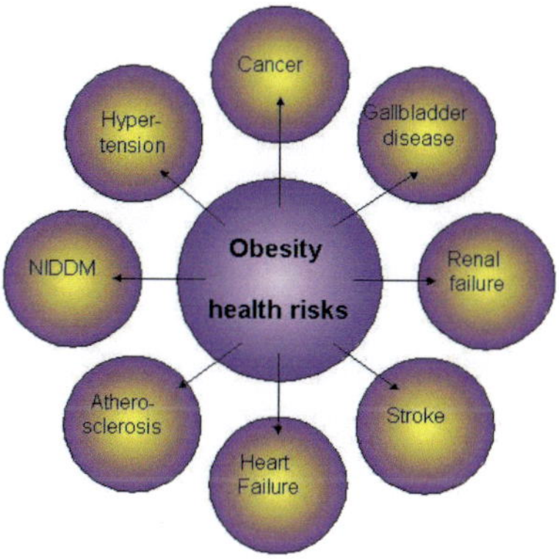

What the "Authorities" Say

National Women's Health Network
A Voice for Women, A Network for Change

Current statistics show that African-American women are five to ten times more likely to develop fibroids than women of other racial groups. Women who are overweight or obese for their height based on body mass index are also at an elevated risk for developing fibroids as compared to women who are an average weight for their height. Research shows that women who have given birth are also at lower risk for developing uterine fibroids.

However, because researchers **don't know what causes fibroids**, it is difficult to decipher all the risk factors.

Black–White Differences in Hysterectomy Prevalence: The CARDIA Study

Julie K. Bower, MPH, Pamela J. Schreiner, PhD, Barbara Sternfeld, PhD, and Cora E. Lewis, MD, MSPH

Black Versus White

Among women who underwent hysterectomy (regardless of oophorectomy status), 78% were Black, whereas only 22% were White. Table 3 compares key participant characteristics by race, pooling women with hysterectomy regardless of oophorectomy status. White women who had undergone hysterectomy with or without oophorectomy had more years of education, lower BMI, lower incidence of tubal ligation, and lower prevalence of self-reported history of fibroids and were more physically active than were Black women who had undergone a hysterectomy ($P < .05$). White women with no history of hysterectomy were on average older, reported older age at menarche, completed more years of schooling, had lower BMI and smaller waist circumference, were less likely to report depressive symptoms, had a lower percentage of smoking history and prior pregnancy, were more likely to drink alcohol at least occasionally, were more physically active, and had lower prevalence of fibroids and self-reported tubal ligation history.

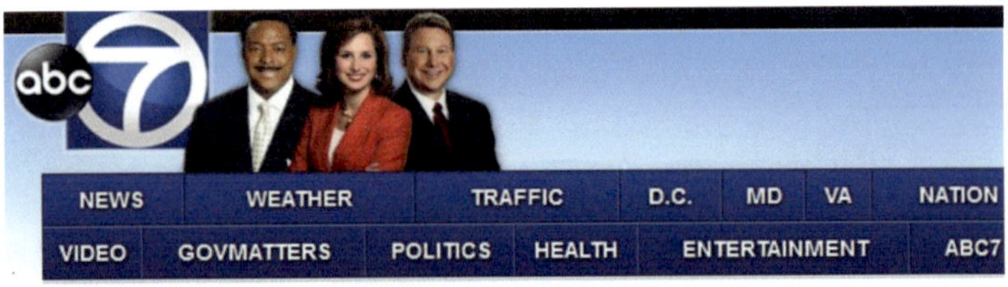

Hot Topics » Fall colors photos | Virginia Governor's Race | LAX shooting | Doug Gansler

HEALTH

African-American women have highest obesity rate: CDC says

December 10, 2012 - 04:30 am

African-American women have the highest obesity rate of any group of Americans. Four out of five black women have a body mass index above 25 percent, the threshold for being overweight or obese, according to the Centers for Disease Control and Prevention. By comparison, nearly two-thirds of Americans overall are in this category, the CDC said.

Historically black, all-female Spelman College in Atlanta is disbanding its NCAA teams and devoting those resources to a campus-wide wellness program. In an open letter announcing Spelman's "wellness revolution," president Beverly Daniel Tatum cited a campus analysis that found many of Spelman's 2,100 students already have high blood pressure, Type 2 diabetes or other chronic ailments.

The Fat Stats

- More than 80% of people with Type-2 Diabetes are overweight
- People who are overweight are more likely to suffer from high blood pressure
- People who are overweight are more likely to suffer from high levels of blood fat
- People who are overweight are more likely to suffer from LDL cholesterol
- All Risk Factors for Heart Disease and Stroke
- In 2010, African Americans were 70% less likely to engage in activity as Non-Hispanic Whites active physical
- Deaths from Heart Disease & Stroke are almost twice the rate for African-Americans as compared to Whites.

THE AFRICAN-AMERICAN MYSTERY SOLVED

It appears that African American women are outright cursed with reproductive diseases and disorders, especially those related to estrogen dominance. African-Americans lead the world in fibroids, endometriosis, and polycystic ovary syndrome (PCOS) with risk factors more than tripling those of other races, and that is at best. The actual statistic for the risk factor of African-American women getting fibroids is 9.7 times as compared to their white counterparts. So, what is the actual cause of this unbelievable disparity?

There are two defining genetic factors that dictate the relationship between African-American women and estrogen. The first is found in the function of their estrogen receptors, and the second within their metabolic system.

Estrogen Receptors

Before we delve into identifying what's different about the way African-American women's estrogen receptors function, it's important to understand what estrogen receptors are, and how they work.

Estrogen receptors are special proteins found within and on the surface of certain cells throughout the body, including but not limited to endometrial, uterine, ovarian and breast cells. The estrogen hormone is distributed through the bloodstream and, classically, diffuses across or into cells where it binds to the estrogen receptor (ER)in the cell nucleus. This initiates a cascade of estrogen response element sequences and protein to protein interactions, which, in a functional reality, play an essential role in the growth and development of female secondary sexual characteristics, such as breasts, pubic and armpit hair, and the regulation of the menstrual cycle and reproductive system. It is also essential in the development of bones, known as osteogenesis.

The ER exists in 2 main forms, ER alpha (ERα) and ER beta (ERβ). ERα and ERβ are encoded by separate genes, Estrogen Receptor 1 (ESR1) and Estrogen Receptor 2 (ESR2), respectively, and have distinct tissue expression patterns. The type of estrogen receptor to which estrogen binds within any given cell determines how sensitive the cell is to the hormone. Upregulation is the increase of sensitivity, when estrogen binds to ERα. Simply put the estrogen is expressed with more potency. Downregulation occurs when estrogen binds to ERβ, which decreases the sensitivity of the cell to estrogen, that is, estrogen becomes weaker. In the cases of fibroids, endometriosis, PCOS and ovarian cysts, uterine, endometrial and ovarian cells become highly sensitive to ingested xenoestrogens, because they upregulate estrogen as it binds prolifically to ERα. The physiological response and result of the amplification of estrogen is inflammation in its many cardinal forms, namely **tumor** (growths/swelling), **dolor** (pain), **rubor** (redness) and **calor** (heat/burning).

So, why are black or African-American women at such a high risk?

The answer is found in the African-American ERα gene expression, as a result of a specific genetic **polymorphism**, which amplifies the function of the receptors. A polymorphism is a variation in the DNA sequence that occurs in a population with a frequency of 1 % or higher. Scientific institutions have historically taught that the higher incidence within a population suggests that a polymorphism is naturally occurring, with either a neutral or beneficial effect. This does not seem to be the case with this particular polymorphism. Polymorphisms are grouped under what are called **genotypes**. In a white paper study entitled **"Ethnic distribution of estrogen receptor-α polymorphism is associated with a higher prevalence of uterine leiomyomas in black Americans"** conducted by the Department of Obstetrics and Gynecology, University of Texas Medical Branch, Galveston, Texas, and published in September, 2006 by the American Society for Reproductive Medicine, the ERα genotype identified as "PP" was found to profoundly increase the risk of leiomyomas (fibroids) and also was directly associated with other severe reproductive diseases. This same **PP** genotype was found to be present in more than 37% of the African-American women just within the study. This percentage is suspected to be even greater among the African-American population. The PP genotype also demonstrated an enhanced estrogen responsiveness in-vitro, meaning it causes greater upregulation, cellular sensitivity and amplification of the effects of estrogen.

Figure 1 below shows how the ER PP genotype excessively multiplies myometrial (uterine muscle) cell proliferation (growth) compared to the pp genotype when exposed to estradiol (E2). This is a controlled environment experimentation example of how fibroid growth differs for each genotype.

FIGURE 1

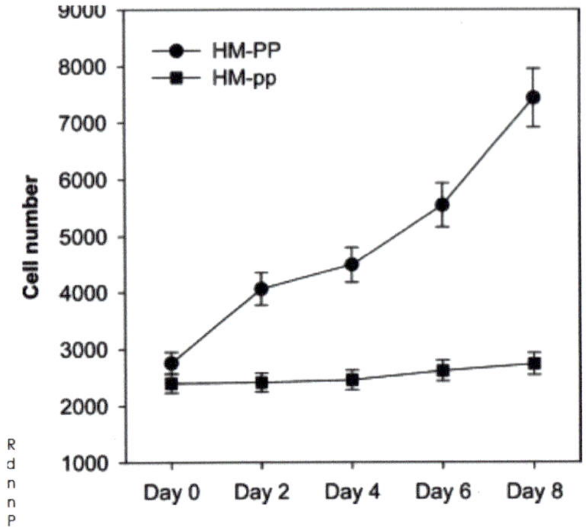

Effect of ER polymorphism on E2-induced proliferation of human myometrial cells. Four human myometrial (HM) cell lines with ER PP genotype (HM 163, HM 188, HM 278, and HM 284) grow significantly faster than four ER pp HM cell lines (HM 97, HM 137, HM 178, and HM 196) (P=.0001). Each value is mean ± SEM of the corresponding cells in two independent experiments.

Al-Hendy. ERA polymorphism and leiomyoma risk. Fertil Steril 2006.

Abnormal Estrogen Metabolism in African-Americans

Metabolism is the sum of the chemical reactions that take place within each cell of a living organism and that provide energy for vital processes and for synthesizing new organic material. Metabolism consists of anabolism (the buildup of substances) and catabolism (the breakdown of substances). The term metabolism is commonly used to refer specifically to the breakdown of food and its transformation into energy. It is the third part of a four-part high-level process:

1. **Ingestion** – the intake of material substances into the body via eating, drinking, breathing, insertion or absorption/injection through the skin.

2. **Digestion** - the process of breaking down food by mechanical and enzymatic action in the alimentary canal/gastrointestinal tract into substances that can be used by the body.

3. **Metabolism** – how the cells utilize the energy we have absorbed from food during digestion

4. **Excretion** – the process of the elimination or expulsion of waste matter from the body

Abnormal estrogen metabolism is a key component of reproductive disorders and diseases in African-American women (and men). It has even been heavily implicated in various cancers, including breast, ovarian, uterine, prostate and kidney cancer. Our focus in this book is the role of abnormal estrogen metabolism and its implications in fibroids, cysts, endometriosis, PCOS, PMS, cramping, amenorrhea and heavy menstrual bleeding.

First, recall that estrogen is derived from androgenic sex hormones, namely testosterone and androstenedione, through a process called aromatization by the enzyme aromatase. In order for estrogen to become "activated" it must pass through the first phase of metabolism, called **hydroxylation**. Hydroxylation is the addition of a hydroxyl group (oxygen and hydrogen) to a metabolized substance. Specific hydroxylated estrogens possess powerful, and potentially harmful effects. These are the very effects that bestow estrogen with its undesirable and cancer-promoting reputation.

The aromatase enzymes that are responsible for the activation and hydroxylation of estrogens are part of the class of enzymes known as CYP450's (cytochrome P450). A sidebar fact to note is that the estrogen hydroxylation enzymes CYP450's are also integral in the metabolism of opioid drugs and toxic chemicals. In fact, the known cancer-promoting effect of certain environmental chemicals is largely due to how these chemicals are hydroxylated via the various CYP450 enzymes.

Hydroxylation is often a volatile process. When a chemical, or when certain estrogens are hydroxylated, they become highly reactive, and prone towards stronger reactions with other molecules, cells and tissues. When there are accelerated levels of hydroxylation activity, there can be havoc, extreme amounts of toxicity in the body, and an increase in the number of serious health problems. A common finding among people with accelerated hydroxylation is chemical sensitivity. For example, such a person smells a chemical and gets nauseous, gets a headache, or some other irritable symptom shows up immediately after. This is usually the case, however, it's not always true for every individual.

CYP450's are a very diverse group of enzymes that depend on genetic coding to determine how they are expressed. Say hello to polymorphism again. Some of the CYP450's are genetically coded (expressed) for "up-regulated" function, while others are coded for "down-regulated" functions. Identifying whether a certain polymorphism encodes for up-regulated (increased) enzyme function, or down-regulated (decreased) enzyme function is absolutely significant, especially with respect to estrogen metabolism. The way genes are expressed in each individual is known as **epigenetics**.

Epigenetics 101

The genes inherited from our parents determine certain characteristics and traits. They also play an important role in determining specific functions within the body. As mentioned above, genes are simply the sequencing of DNA. Epigenetics affects how those genes are read and expressed by your cells which, in turn, determines how they produce said essential and crucial proteins.

The functionality of epigenetics is best described as follows:

- It regulates genes, enabling some to be inactive or expressed – genes that are switched off remain dormant while genes that are switched on are active.

- It is everywhere – in your diet, in the air you breathe, your exercise regimen (or the lack thereof), when and how much you sleep – and it can cause chemical alterations to the genes, causing them to switch off over time.

- It is the very thing that makes you unique – the combination of specific genes that are switched on or off determines your exclusive qualities such as hair and eye color, and all your other physical traits.

- It is technically reversible – with an unlimited number of combinations for genes being switched on or off, solving and then mastering how to reverse a gene's state could lead to the intracellular cures for cancer, obesity, and other chronic diseases.

If you're still having a challenge coming to terms with understanding the what and how behind the nature and mechanics of epigenetics the following analogy will definitely help:

Imagine that a person's lifespan is a movie. The cast of actors and actresses are the cells, making up the fundamental units of the movie.

Their DNA is the script, providing the essential instructions for how the cells (actors and actresses) perform their respective assigned roles. The individual DNA sequences (genes) are the story/lines/words of the script with certain blocks of words providing instructions that determine the actions and events taking place in the living body (movie).

In this analogy, genetics is basically the act of screenwriting, whereas epigenetics is the task and role of directing. The director receives a specific script, but he has the aptitude and power to change and/or eliminate entire scenes or merely pieces of dialogue which will have an overall effect on the whole, for better or for worse. So, in essence your epigenetics – your environment, your diet, your exercise regimen, your sleep patterns – can direct your health to either be the best it can possibly be, or it can be a rotten tomato - rife with a succession of acute, chronic or even fatal health conditions. Is it a little clearer now?

There is a second phase of estrogen metabolism, which is referred to as the "inactivation" phase. This phase 2 reaction is **Methylation**. Methylation is essential in the process of detoxification of chemicals, xenobiotics, drugs and, in the interest of this book, steroid hormones such as estrogen. Methylation of estrogen is a major mechanism that blocks the toxic effects of estrogen from causing DNA damage. When a methyl molecule group substitutes or is tacked onto a hydroxylated estrogen it actually neutralizes the hydroxylation effects. Certain methylated estrogens even show protective and anti-inflammatory effects on cells. It is important to note, however, that due to the vast complexities of the human genome, there are certain DNA segments called "promoter regions" where methylation may initiate or contribute to cancer through a process known as hypermethylation.

African-American/Black women share an affinity of polymorphism at the CYP19A1 gene that exacerbates hydroxylation, and diminishes methylation. This results in the upregulation of the CYP19A1 gene, which is the specific CYP450 that encodes aromatase, the enzyme responsible for converting androgens to estrogens. Numerous studies have concluded that the up-regulation of CYP19A1 is correlated with the pathogenesis of leiomyoma (fibroid) tumors. One such study by Hiroshi Ishikawa et al, published in The

Journal of Clinical Endocrinology & Metabolism, Volume 94, Issue 5, 1 May 2009, Pages 1752–1756, found an 83-fold amount of aromatase mRNA levels in fibroid tissue compared with adjacent myometrium in African-American women. This is the exact reason why fibroids occur more frequently and at an earlier age in African-American women. All such studies have shown that African-American women exhibit much higher CYP19A1 mRNA levels in fibroids than all other populations.

FIGURE 2

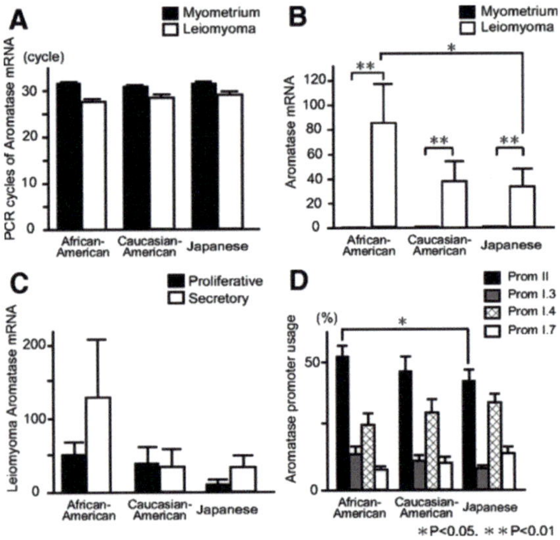

Expression of aromatase mRNA and promoter (Prom) usage in uterine leiomyomas of African-American, Caucasian-American, and Japanese women

Double-Whammy

It is the combination of these specific polymorphisms - the first at the estrogen receptor level, and the second at the metabolism of the enzyme aromatase – that has resulted in the pandemic of reproductive diseases and conditions that is afflicting black women absolutely everywhere on the planet. This is the very reason why we implore and beseech all black women to refrain from the dietary habits that are practiced by other races.

OUR HERELIMINATION™ KIT (AND PROGRAM) IS THE SOLUTION TO ERADICATE THESE STATISTICS

CHAPTER 6

The Fibroid Elimination Bible Program

The Program Consists of 3 Distinct Phases:

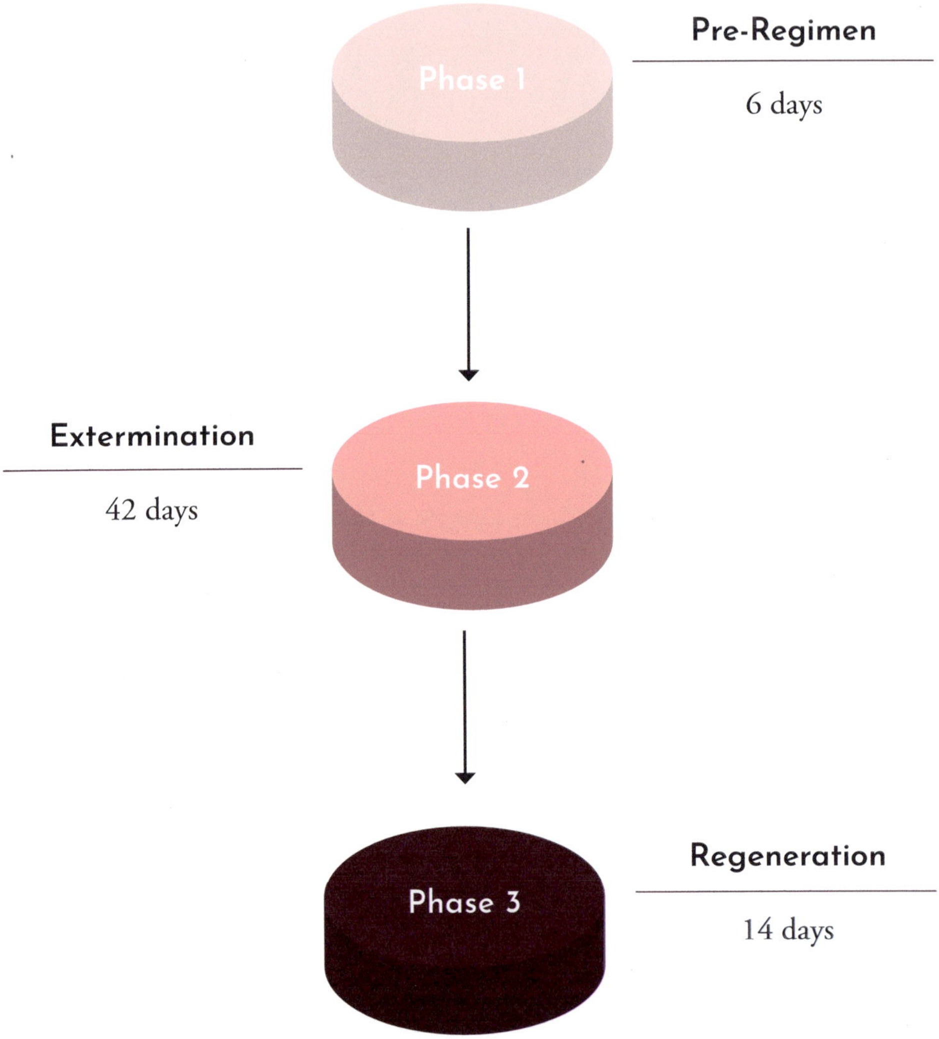

Phase 1: Pre-Regimen 6 days

The Pre-Regimen phase is an intermediary stage which briskly ushers and prepares your body for the Extermination phase. It is much like the stretching an athlete does before starting a game, or the warm-up you do before a workout. It is the phase of weaning you off your current diet, over the 6-day period, while introducing the specialized eHealth Fibroid Elimination Diet. You may begin supplementing your diet with all the HerElimination™ supplements to cleanse and rebuild your red blood cells and lymph, whilst obliterating that superfluous white adipose tissue.

Phase 2: Extermination 42 days

The Extermination phase is where we buckle down to business and aggressively starve your fibroids of their food supply. During this stage your pre-existing eating habits MUST be completely quashed – they are the source and root cause of your condition, and the eHealth Fibroid Elimination Diet will be your sole source of nutrition. he Essence™ Fibroid Formula elixir will be introduced at this stage to annihilate your unwanted guests. In this phase you will be implementing your strict exercise regimen. This is a combination of aerobic exercises and Qi-gong exercises, specifically targeting key meridians (neurons, smooth muscle groups, organs and glands) of your body that have either suffered or atrophied as a result of your condition. It is imperative that you keep up with our regimen to, not only expedite results, but to re-energize and sculpt your body into its true and beautiful shape.

Phase 3: Regeneration 14

The Regeneration phase is an extension of the Extermination phase, but it is slightly less focused on extermination and more focused on energizing, strengthening and rebuilding muscle tissue that may have diminished during phase 2. An increase in food intake along with the dietary supplements will guarantee the desired results. An increase in repetitions within your exercise regimen will also contribute greatly in achieving your goal.

CHAPTER 7

electric pHood™ Dietary Supplements

The only way to guarantee and achieve the exact results that you desire, is to provide your body with the exact minerals, and nutrient content, that will target, detoxify, feed and repair specific cells, tissues, organs and systems.

The electric pHood™ elixir formulas are the nucleus of the HerElimination™ Kit. Your obtaining of these products is an absolute prerequisite for this program.

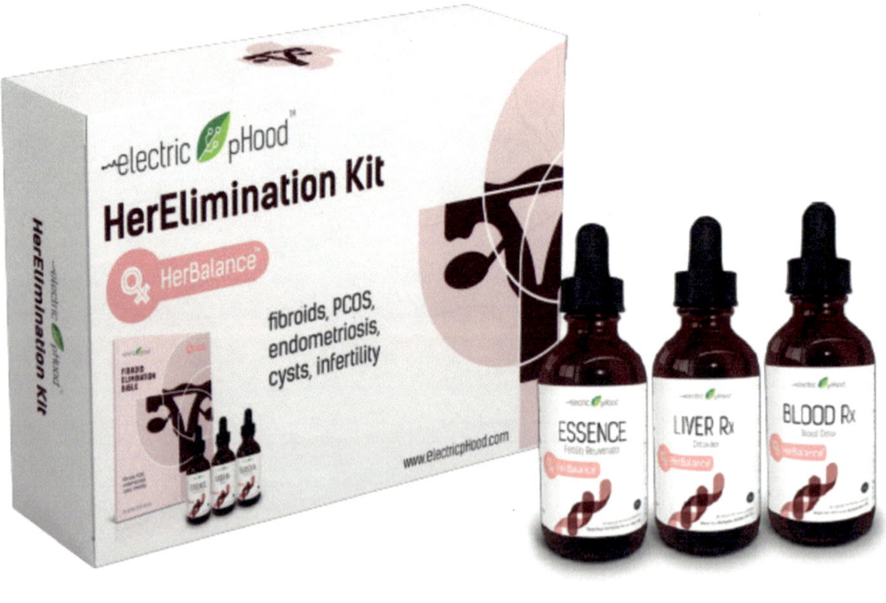

Nature's pHarmacy

Essence™

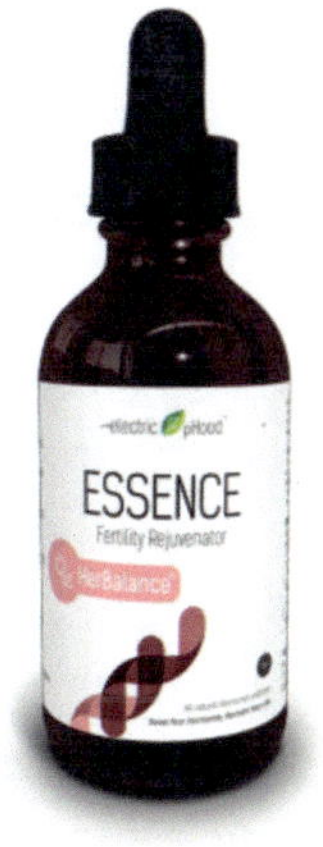

An indigenous antibacterial, antifungal, antiviral, and anti-inflammatory female reproductive health and hormone stimulating/stabilizing fibroid & cyst formula, used to support the body in eliminating ovarian, uterine and sexually transmitted diseases, and to amplify libido.

Blood Rx™

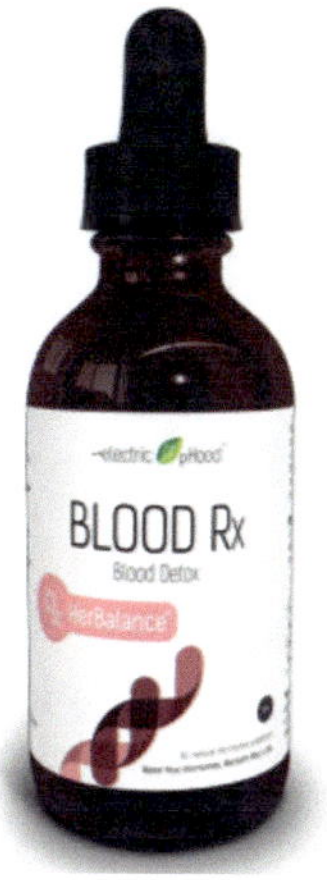

An indigenous antibacterial, antifungal, antiviral, anti-inflammatory blood and lymphatic electric charger, and detoxifying formula, used to eliminate all parasites and adverse microbes from all cells, tissues and organs, throughout the entire body.

Liver Rx™

The World's most powerful autoimmune disorder and liver disorder elimination supporting formula. An antibacterial, antifungal, antiviral, and anti -carcinogenic formula made to support the body to neutralize leukocytes, and reverse Arthritis, Gout, Diabetes I & II, Hepatitis and Lupus. This formula contains the Earth's MOST MAGNETIC minerals that contain octahedral and hexagonal based carbon molecules which provide the highest cell and tissue regenerative power on the planet.

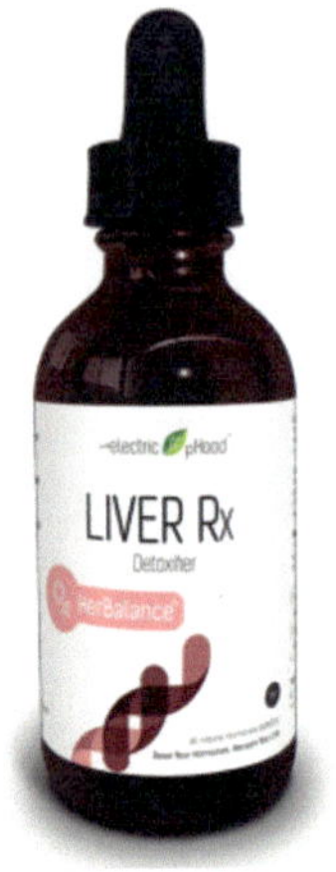

Eliminate™

If your fibroids or cysts are larger than 3cm across any dimension, or you have 4 or more of the former or latter, then we recommend that you to add Eliminate to your dietary supplements to provide the body with the necessary nutrients for it to expedite your elimination process.

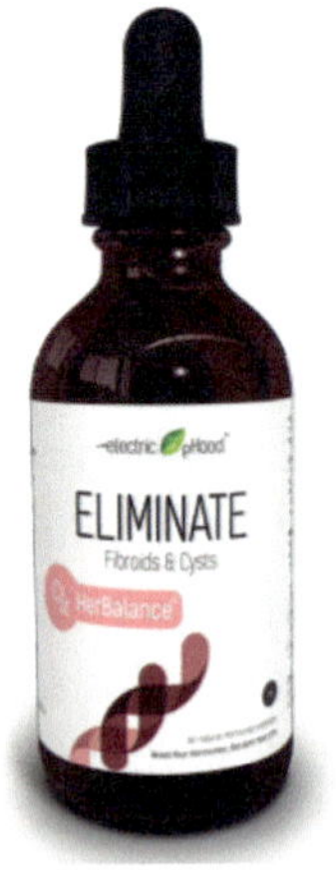

CHAPTER 8

Phase 1: Pre-Regimen

Let's jump right in with "your" diet – the perpetrator and absolute culprit of your condition. Diet, by eHealth's definition, is any and all substances that one intakes and/or ingests into one's body. This means it is not only bad food that is responsible for your ailing health, but the air you breathe (your environment), and the lack of sunlight – the sole source of your vitamin D. As relocation is not a mandate of this manual, we will forgive your environment (for now) and focus on your food and daily exposure to sunlight.

It is not our intention to pull any punches with the Fibroid Elimination Bible. You have exactly one week to give up ALL of the following foods:

- Alfalfa
- Anise
- Antacids
- Anti-Depressants***
- Baker's Yeast***
- Barley
- Caffeine
- Eggplant
- Red Beans
- Clover
- Condiments***
- Cowpeas (Black-eyed Peas)
- Dairy Foods***
- Eggs
- Eggplant
- Fennel
- Fermented Food***
- Flaxseeds***
- Garlic
- Hops (all Beer and Alcohol)***
- Licorice
- Olives
- Papaya
- Parsley
- Peas
- Bell Peppers
- Pomegranate
- Potatoes (white)
- Pumpkin
- Red Beans
- Red Clover
- Rhubarb
- Rice (Brown/White)
- Sage
- Sesame Seeds (white)
- Soybean Sprouts***
- Soybeans***
- Soybean Oil***
- Sunflower Seeds***

- Wheat***
- Yam
- All Purines
- Plastic Bottle Water
- Frozen/Thawed
- Neglected Water
- ALL ANIMAL

***Most adverse foods

Now…it should be clarified at this point that not all the foods listed above are "bad", generally speaking, but are foods that do, however, contribute, in varying degrees, to your exogenous estrogen supply. The temporary elimination of all the foods above, we call an "Estrogen Fast". Once your fibroids have been totally eliminated you may reintroduce only the foods from this list that have beneficial properties to your health, for example, Dates, Cucumbers and Cherries (organic only).

Condiments are the silent killers. Most so-called "healthy eaters" who haphazardly apply these sides to their dishes, don't realize the immense damage that sauces, such as ketchup, hot sauce and mayonnaise, inflict upon their systems. They are riddled with neurotoxins, glutamates, yeasts and sugar. Condiments should be omitted at all costs

Dude, What the Hell am I Supposed to Eat?

You are not the first, and certainly won't be the last to express this exact sentiment, but rest assured we have you covered.

CHAPTER 9

eHealth Diet Classifications

Your health is ultimately determined by your self-discipline, or the lack thereof. The old adage "it's only a sin once you know it's wrong", is our mantra in self-discipline. Knowledge is power and key to how you "choose" to eat to live. The following paragraphs will provide you with enough information for you to correctly categorize your present and future dietary lifestyles:

First you MUST understand *exactly* what "food" is. According to eHealth:-

Food is any living nutritional part of a plant that interfaces with the human body and adds vitality and energy, and sustains health physically, mentally and spiritually. Food adds phototropic Sun and plant based: 1) negative hydrogen ions, 2) oxygen, 3) water, 4) carbon and other minerals, as fuel for the body. In a nutshell, food is bio-available carbohydrates from plants.

Baring eHealth's definition of food in mind, the following will make perfect sense.

Class F Diet - The "Suicide" Diet"

The Class F Diet includes the ingestion of any type of Drugs, on top of the Flesh and Starch Diet of Class E. This includes smoking weed, the taking of prescription pills and/or medication, and all other syrup related drugs. This is the epitome of a destructive and habitual diet that is commonly associated with emotionally unstable individuals, who are in dire need of an eHealth clinic. Contrary to the justifiers' belief, smoking weed is NOT healthy. The **cannabinoids** (the chemical compounds with medicinal properties) are concentrated in the seeds, and are carbohydrates that should only be either eaten or made into a tea for consumption. Smoking the leaves or buds produces high levels of ammonia and ammonium cyanide in the lungs, blocking the lung alveoli which, in turn, reduce the necessary amount of oxygen to the brain.

Tetrahydrocannabinol, or THC, the cannabinoid constituent responsible for the "high" is a highly psychoactive chemical, which has been strongly linked to psychosis. In natural/wild cannabis THC represents between only 0.1 and 1.0 percent of the total constituency of the plant, and its counterpart cannabidiol or CBD, which is an antipsychotic, is as high as 10 percent. The problem lies in the extremely high amount of THC in the new GMO strains where THC can be as high as 65 percent, which diminishes the constituent percentage of CBD and other useful cannabinoids. For this reason we strongly advise you to not partake in weed smoking before, during or after your elimination.

Class E Diet – Flesh & Starch

We at eHealth call this the "Genesis 9 Diet" of the heterotrophic nations. This diet is filled with animal fat, which is COMPLETELY indigestible by herbivores (natural plant eaters).

Animal fat creates white fat, aka white adipose tissue, in the body, which ferments into white blood cells, which have the ultimate goal of parasitically eating your blood and melanin.

There is absolutely no nutrition in flesh. There is, however, traces of the remnant waste of the plants which the poor animal ate before being slaughtered, if it was, at all, allowed to even graze. **All disease** is caused by this poor diet of flesh and starch, which is evidenced by the terrible, foul odor that is released with defecation. This foul odor is indicative of the inner fermentation and rotting of internal digestive organs. This IS the disease diet.

Class D Diet – The "Starchatarian" Diet

eHealth coined the term ***Starchatarian*** to describe one who partakes in the idle diet of overcooked veganism. Starchatarians are those people who profess to be vegetarians or vegans, but overcook and kill their would-be living food and then digest the substance wastes, which are nothing but toxic starches. This is also known as the **confusion diet**, simply because the consumer believes that he or she is eating healthy but in actuality isn't, and becomes just as sick as one indulging in a Class E (or even a Class F) diet. Upon the realization that the misguided diet is somewhat useless, these individuals resort back to flesh and starch, proclaiming to the world and its uncle that vegetarianism and veganism does not work.

Another prime example of a Starchatarian is your classic "rice and beans" eater.

This deadly combination of grain and legume has crept its way into almost all post-colonialist, indigenous cultures and has wreaked havoc in its wake. Rice is riddled with nasty little bacteria called **Bacillus Cereus**. This is the bacterium that is responsible for harmful food poisoning conditions, such as **Fried Rice Syndrome**, which is the result of the spores multiplying when rice is left sitting at room temperature for long periods of time before consumption. All beans contain the symbionts, rhizobium bacteria and mycorrhizal fungi, which are nitrogen fixators, meaning they absorb nitrogen gas and convert it into ammonium compounds. Your body is always trying to rid itself of nitrogen, and its derivatives, primarily through your liver, as it is a poison. Eating beans or most grains without thoroughly soaking (neutralizing the nitrogen) in water is a guaranteed way to cause damage in the intestines and an increase in fermentation (rotting). Fermentation produces alcohol… and whoops we're back to Class F!!!

Class C Diet – electric Vegans & Vegetarians Diet

This is the first stage of actual healthy eating. This is the practice of eating only organic and wild fruits, organic and wild vegetables, and organic and wild grains. That is, none of the food is grown conventionally (sprayed with pesticides). Pesticides destroy the glandular and endocrine system of the body, escalate cancerous estrogens, and alter nerve signaling, via their dense ammonium compounds.

On the Class C Diet, one never cooks fruits or vegetables. The only "light" cooking is performed on grains (after thorough soaking in water) like the master grain Quinoa, Amaranth and Black/Wild Rice. Overcooking plants destroys their atomic vitality. In fact, plants never need to be cooked. They can, rather, be soaked in hot water to tenderize; time depending upon the plant. This class employs the use of dehydrators to make non- cooked dishes such as cakes, pies, cookies, kale chips, etc., without killing the food.

Class B Diet – electric Raw Food Diet

This is a strict diet where the practitioner only partakes in the consumption of raw fruits and raw vegetables. There are absolutely zero cooked or dehydrated ingredients in any and all dishes. Again, the fruits and vegetables are organic and/or wild. Produce is either bought at farmers' markets or grown by the practitioner. Plant cells perform the task of replacing/replenishing weak or depleted body cells through the process of firstly being converted into erythrocytes (red blood cells) in the intestines, and then being assigned by the liver to the specific cells, organs or glands.

Class A Diet – electric Fruitarian Diet

This is the diet of eternal youth and perpetual health. The practitioner only eats seeded organic or wild fruits, which provide only carbohydrates and glucose, the quintessential fuel of the body. Remove the skin and the seeds of all fruits before consumption for optimum results.

CHAPTER 10

Food Substitutions & Replacements

It is imperative that we again emphasize that the Blood Rx™ and Liver Rx™ medicinal mineral and nutritive blends are an integral part of this program and MUST be used in conjunction with the transitional food regimen. This will allow the medicinal properties to activate your inherent self-healing functions much more efficiently; considering that the imbalanced composition of foods created the environment that obstructed normal functioning, homeostasis and self healing, thereby creating the need for medicinal plant therapy.

A transitional (Class C)food regimen that swiftly decreases aromatase (exogenous estrogens) intake is imperative; it entails the principle of substitution to expeditiously transition from refined complex (wheat) carbohydrates to unrefined non-wheat grains, and a transition from high-starch vegetables to low-starch and high carbohydrate vegetables.

Eliminate **meat** from your diet from "Day One". ALL meats contain, among a host of other parasites, **prions**. Prions are infectious protein particles that replicate by assimilating/devouring, primarily, brain tissue, and are not only the cause of neurological degenerative diseases, such as Creutzfeldt-Jakob Disease (CJD), but are impossible (thus far) to eliminate/cure.

- **Wheat (gluten)** is by far the most detrimental grain in existence; just as wheat based foods are the most detrimental of grain based foods. They are the most contributive to fibroids, diabetes, weight gain and obesity, and should be of a priority measure for substitution.

- **Quinoa** on the contrary has the lowest carb (glycemic) levels of all grains in existence, and is the most appropriate substitute for all adverse grains.

- **Wild rice (black)** is the original rice species (grass seed) that is presently wild crafted in Minnesota and Wisconsin. Its starch complexity is more digestible than brown, basmati and especially white rice (which are mutant descendants of wild rice)

- **Butternut and bush scallop squash (steamed or baked)** are the perfect substitute for root vegetable species of potatoes, turnips and rutabagas; their starch content is of a much lesser degree.

SUBSTITUTIONS	
FUTURE	PAST
Quinoa Quinoa/Millet/Teff/	Wheat Couscous/Rice/Grits/
Amaranth/Spelt Wild Rice (black)	Oatmeal Rice: white or brown
Butternut/Acorn Squash	Potatoes/Turnips/Rutabagas
Scallions/Red Onions	White Onions
Chives	Garlic
Green-Snap/Black Navy Beans	Kidney/Black-eyed/White/Baked Beans
Olmec (Mexican) Wild Blue Corn	Yellow Corn
Sweet Peppers	Bell Peppers
Quinoa/Spelt/Millet Spaghetti/ Pasta	Wheat Spaghetti/Pasta

As amazing as we are at eHealth, we are neither able to remotely detect, nor speculate upon all the forbidden foods of which you are currently partaking yet😉 but the table above should sufficiently cover your general staple(transitional) diet.

Another important factor for us to point out, at this junction, is how you should prepare your meals. Below is a comparative Dos & Don'ts list, to which you must adhere to guarantee the best results on your journey.

DON'Ts

Fry - to cook food in, or on the surface of, an extremely hot grease solution. This destroys all its vital components.

Barbecue - to grill food over a toxic, charcoal-based fire.

Boil - to cook food in boiling water; this devitalizes most nutrients and transfers the others into the water solution.

Saute' - to fry on the surface of a pan with small amounts of oil, at a moderately hot temperature.

DOs

Bake - to cook in an oven at low or medium temperatures.

Simmer – to heat foods below the boiling point at the lowest possible fire setting.

Steam - to prepare food in a pot with holes at the bottom, that's placed within another pot filled with water, forcing steam upward partially cooking food.

Marinate - to immerse a vegetable food into a liquid solution for a certain period of time

New Diet = New Lifestyle

Below is the eHealth Lifestyle Food List. These are the foods that you can eat for the rest of your life, during and after you obliterate those fibroids, which will ensure your optimum health. We have made this list as extensive as possible, but you can also research the nutritional benefits of other foods to add to your list as you become more experienced in the healthy lifestyle.

- Acorn Squash
- Almonds
- Amaranth
- Artichoke
- Basil
- Blackberries
- Black Kale (Dinosaur)*
- Black Lentils
- Black Mulberries
- Black Rice
- Blueberries
- Broccoli *
- Brussels Sprouts
- Burdock
- Butternut Squash
- Chard
- Chives
- Chlorophyll
- Coconuts
- Collard Greens
- Dandelion

- Dates*
- Fenugreek
- Figs
- Forbidden Black Rice
- Ginger
- Goji Berries
- Grape Tomatoes
- Grapefruits
- Green Cabbage
- Green or Purple Pears
- Hemp Seeds
- Lemons
- Limes / Key Limes
- Mangoes
- Millet
- Mustard Greens
- Pineapples
- Purple Cabbage
- Purple Seeded Grapes
- Quinoa (Black/Red)
- Raw Pumpkin Seeds
- Red Musa Bananas
- Red Onions
- Roma Tomatoes
- Romaine Lettuce
- Seaweed (Nori)
- Seaweed (Wakame)
- Seaweed (Arame)
- Spelt
- Tuna Plant
- Water (Distilled)
- Water (Spring)
- Water (Structured)
- Watermelon
- Wild Raspberries
- Wild Rice
- Wild Yam
- Yellow Squash
- Zucchini Squash

CHAPTER 11

The Pre-Regimen Diet

6 DAYS

Eat 3 solid meals a day, substituting your usual ingredients with the above-mentioned ingredients gradually until your dysfunctional diet has been totally replaced (by Day 6). Alternatively, you can begin phasing in our recipes. Simply find recipes you like from our recipe section, and plan out your daily meals for the next six days.

Remember, the more processed foods, meat, coffee, alcohol and dairy you've consumed in the past years, the more toxins your body will have accumulated. Diving right into the Extermination without giving yourself a chance to adjust to the Regimen

Diet can cause extra stress on the body. Doing the Pre-Regimen sends a preparatory signal to your body that positive shifts and bio-chemical changes are about to take place.

Your Biological Clock & Diet:

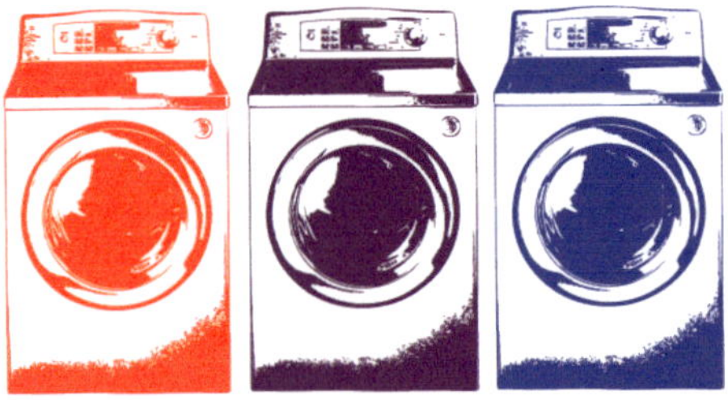

If you've ever heard the phrase, "there's a right time for everything" then you can bet you're your bottom dollar that, when it comes to correct dietary practice, there is no exception. Your body goes through 3 eight-hour biological food processing cycles per day, which are synchronized with the movement and position/absence of the sun. This is a major process of what is called the Circadian Rhythm and it is divided as follows:

- Appropriation Cycle
- Assimilation Cycle
- Elimination Cycle

Appropriation Cycle - eating & digestion

During the hours between 12PM and

8PM, your body is in the Appropriation Cycle. During this period, we are most awake, active, present and therefore efficient at digesting, metabolizing and burning through the majority of our heavily concentrated foods. This is why the majority of meals (lunch, dinner and snacks) also occur during this cycle Eating after 8pm interrupts and impedes the physical process of the **Assimilation Cycle**.

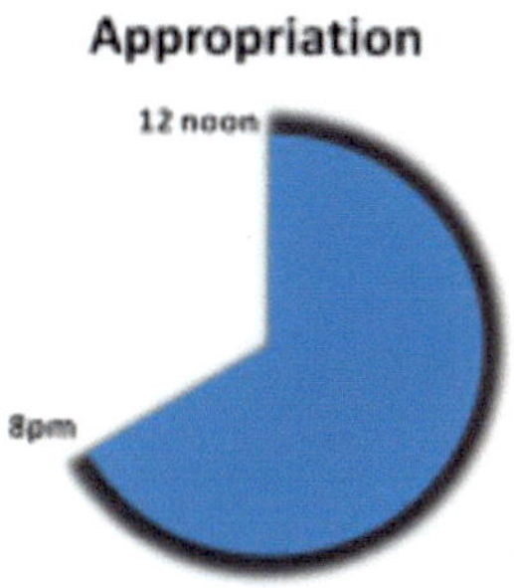

Assimilation Cycle - absorption & use

During the hours between 8PM and 4AM, your body is in the Assimilation Cycle. This is the time you are most likely to be relaxed or sleeping. This period is when all the 'assimilating' or absorbing of nutrients and minerals from your food occurs and gets transported to your organs, bones and cells via the blood. All the rebuilding, renewing and healing take place here. Again, it is best to eat well before this period, so that the foods are digested and out of the stomach. If you continue to eat during this period your body will not utilize the nutrients as they will not be properly processed.

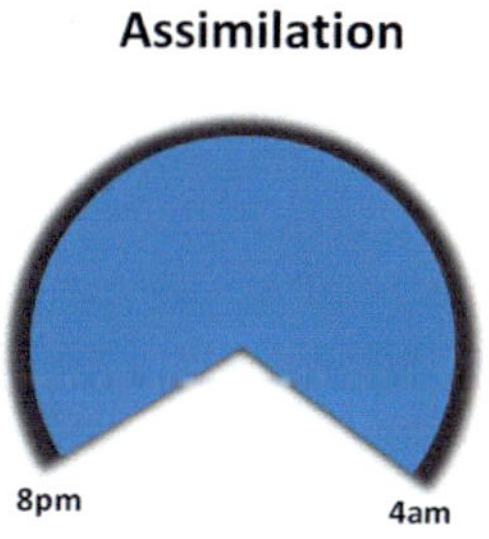

Elimination Cycle - body waste

During the hours between 4AM and12PM, your body is in the Elimination Cycle. It never stops to work on your digestion and you can still eat or drink at this time, but understanding that this is the period most important for cleansing and releasing toxins ('Eliminating'), you must make the right food choices if you are going to eat. It is imperative to stick to liquids and the most hydrating living foods, as you let your body shed the toxins (think how you sometimes wake up feeling tired, sweaty, slight headache, and with bad breath - all are symptoms of detoxing).

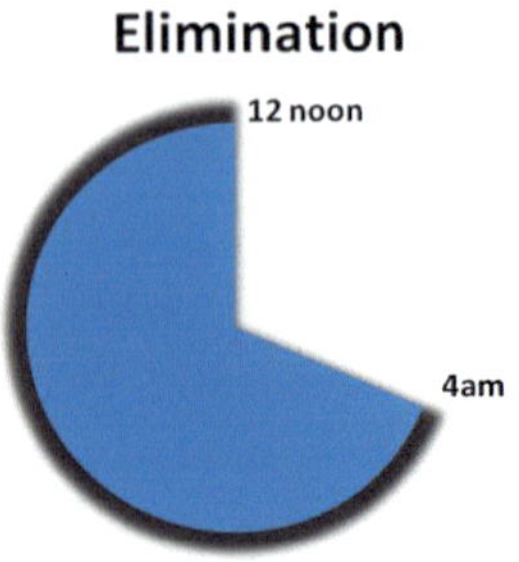

NB: ***If you do not experience complete or healthy elimination of your foods, i.e., sweating, regular urination, and regular defecation, certain organ failure is imminent. Under-arm antiperspirants are known to block the lymph nodes from draining properly, which often causes lumps and tumors in the breasts.***

Most diets that are unsuccessful, or that do not yield desired results, are directly due to inappropriate or irregular eating times that conflict with, or disrupt the circadian rhythm. The Fibroid Elimination Bible program places you on the most efficient path to success, by adhering to the dictates of your body's built-in biological clock.

On a Class A diet, the circadian rhythm does not apply, as the body is essentially metabolizing glucose and carbohydrates that will be efficiently processed by the cells.

Your Phase 1 Daily Diet Plan

7am – 9am	12pm – 2pm	5pm – 7pm	9pm – 10pm
Breakfast	**Lunch**	**Dinner**	**Opt. Snack**
Fruits or Smoothie	Transitional Food	Transitional Food	Fruits or Smoothie
+ Elixirs	**+ Elixirs**	**+ Elixirs**	

Breakfast

Fruit Smoothie

Blend a smoothie with your own choice of ingredients from the eHealth Lifestyle Food List. Examples are almond or coconut milk, additional mineral sources, like nut butters, a hearty amount of greens, like black kale or chard, and moderate amounts of fruit.

Elixirs

Squeeze ½ vial of Essence directly under the tongue.

Squeeze ½ vial of Blood Rx directly under the tongue.

Squeeze ½ vial of Liver Rx directly under the tongue.

Lunch

Transitional Meal

Prepare a hearty solid meal substituting as many ingredients from the SUBSTITUTIONS list, whilst totally eliminating all meat entrees in which you would normally indulge. This is your main meal. Get the most out of it by adding dark green leafy vegetables, and a grain, such as quinoa, for your protein.

Elixirs

Squeeze ½ vial of Essence directly under the tongue.

Squeeze ½ vial of Blood Rx directly under the tongue.

Squeeze ½ vial of Liver Rx directly under the tongue.

Dinner

Transitional Light Meal

Prepare a light meal with as many substitute ingredients as possible, whilst making sure that the meal is, in its majority, a water-based one, like a soup. It is important in this phase that you begin to wean yourself off the traditional heavy meal in the evening. This rationed approach is for the sole purpose of allowing your assimilation cycle to perform its job most efficiently. Digestion of hard and heavy foods utilizes approximately

70% of the body's energy resources, so by eating large portions so close to the assimilation cycle diminishes its nutrient retention rate/ absorption potential immensely.

Elixirs

Squeeze ½ vial of Essence directly under the tongue.

Squeeze ½ vial of Blood Rx directly under the tongue.

Squeeze ½ vial of Liver Rx directly under the tongue.

CHAPTER 12

Phase 1 Exercise Regimen

As stated previously, this phase is focused more on weaning than anything else, but just as an athlete must warm up before engaging in sport, so must you, with a light daily workout. This is a necessary part of your preparation as we want to get your lymphatic fluids active for the ejection of all those parasites and toxins you've been harboring.

Squats: 10 repetitions x 3 sets (add 3 reps per day)

- Stand with your head facing forward and your chest held up and out, with arms by your sides.
- Place your feet shoulder-width apart or slightly position A.
- Sit back and down like you're sitting into an wider to assume imaginary chair, extending and raising your arms to a 90 degree angle in front of you.
- Keep your back as perpendicular as possible.
- Lower down so your thighs are as parallel to the floor as possible, with your knees over your ankles. Press your weight back into your heels assuming position B
- Keep your body tight, and push through your heels to bring yourself back to starting position A

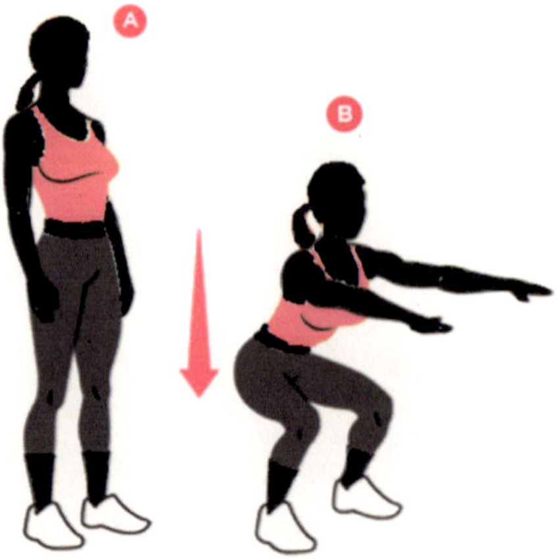

Jumping Jacks: 15 repetitions x 3 sets (add 3 reps per day)

- Stand with feet together, knees slightly bent, and arms to sides. (A)
- Jump while raising arms and separating legs to sides.
- Land on forefoot with legs apart and arms overhead. (B)
- Jump again while lowering arms and returning legs to midline.
- Land on forefoot with arms and legs in original position and repeat.
- Intensity can be increased by jumping faster.

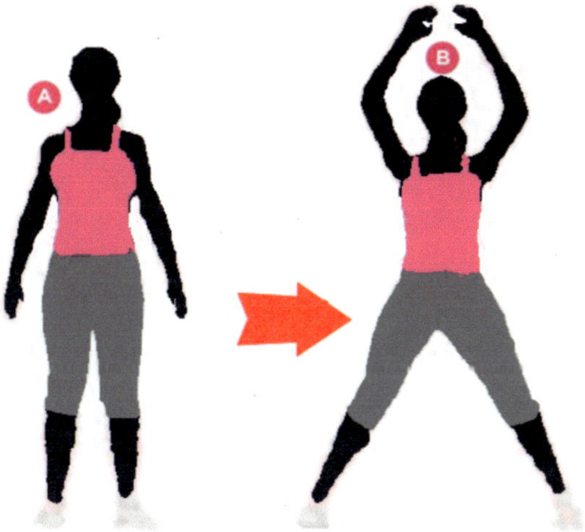

CHAPTER 13

Phase 1 Exercise Calendar

	DAY 1	DAY 2	DAY 3	DAY 4	DAY 5	DAY 6
7AM	SQUATS	JUMPING JACKS	SQUATS	JUMPING JACKS	SQUATS	JUMPING JACKS
1PM	JUMPING JACKS	SQUATS	JUMPING JACKS	SQUATS	JUMPING JACKS	SQUATS
8PM	SQUATS & JUMPING JACKS	SQUATS & JUMPING JACKS	SQUATS & JUMPING JACKS	SQUATS & JUMPING JACKS	SQUATS & JUMPING JACKS	SQUATS & JUMPING JACKS

CHAPTER 14

Phase 2: Fibroid Extermination

You've done the warm up…you've done the stretch…now for the main event!!!

By now you should have weaned yourself, somewhat, off your delinquent diet and replaced your typical foods with those exhibited in the eHealth Lifestyle Food List.

THE EXTERMINATION DIET (CLASS A)

42 DAYS

Eat 3 meals a day, with an additional and specific eHealth night cap, using ONLY FRUITS selected from the eHealth Lifestyle Food List. There are no alternatives.

Your Phase 2 Daily Diet Plan

8am – 11am	12pm – 3pm	5pm – 7pm	9pm – 10pm
Breakfast	**Lunch**	**Dinner**	**Opt. Snack**
Lemon & Fruit Smoothie	Class A Dish	Class A Dish	Lemon
+ Elixirs	**+ Elixirs**	**+ Elixirs**	**+ Elixirs**

Breakfast

Lemon & Smoothie Recipe

Start your day with a fresh organic lemon, squeezing the juice directly under your tongue, followed by eating the whole pulp. This will infuse essential negatively charged ions directly into your bloodstream. This is done prior to your first daily exercise regimen. After your workout be sure to drink a thick fruit smoothie made from ingredients from the eHealth Lifestyle Food List.

Elixirs

Squeeze ½ vial of Essence directly under the tongue.

Squeeze ½ vial of Blood Rx directly under the tongue.

Squeeze ½ vial of Liver Rx directly under the tongue.

Lunch

Main Meal

This should be your heaviest meal of the day. Select your combination of fruits from the eHealth Lifestyle Food List. Again, this is your main and most essential meal. The timing is directly in tune with your natural appropriation cycle, so that it is fully digested well before the initiation of the assimilation cycle. It is important for us to stress that this is not a weight loss diet, even though, during this phase, you are guaranteed to lose weight.

To this end, we strongly recommend that you eat large enough meals to ensure the right amount of essential glucose and carboxylic acids to develop and maintain muscle mass, strength and vitality.

Elixirs

Squeeze ½ vial of Essence of Fertility directly under the tongue.

Squeeze ½ vial of Blood Rx directly under the tongue.

Squeeze ½ vial of Liver Rx directly under the tongue.

Dinner

Light Dinner

Prepare a raw fruit meal from the eHealth Lifestyle Food List. It is most effective if this meal is a lighter than the lunch meal, and a water-based one. Whilst saving energy that would usually be consumed by the digestion of a traditional heavy meal, this approach will maintain your cellular integrity. In its most efficient and healthiest state, the human cell has the following composition:

75% - 85% water

- 3% – 5% carbohydrates – glucose (simple form)
- 12% - 14% carboxylic acids
- 4% structural acids
- 1% - 3% fat

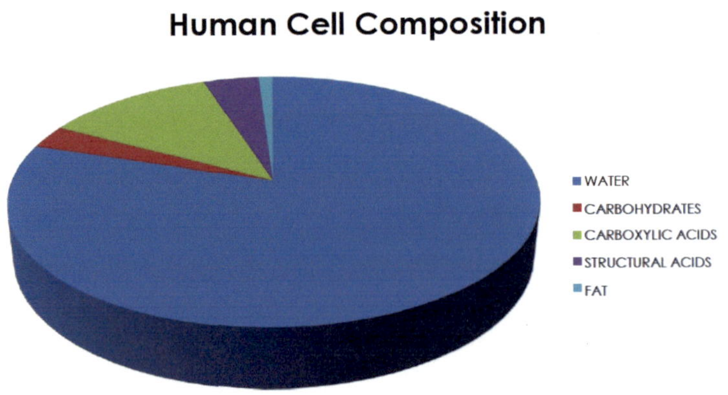

The composition of food types of a typical vegan diet are represented in the table below:

FOOD	WATER	PROTEIN	CARBOHY-DRATES	FAT
	R	N	S	T
Fruits	87%	0.9%	5%	0.7%
Vegetables	80%	2.0%	3%	0.8%
Vegetables (low-starch)	**70%**	2.8%	**9%**	0.4%
Vegetables (high-starch)	**63%**	1.8%	**30%**	0.6%
Grains	**11%**	**8%**	**75%**	0.7%

In an observation of the illustrations, you can clearly see the comparison between the various levels and forms in the **bold** and **underlined** food sectors, and their inconsistency with those of human cell composition, just as you can observe the same levels and forms in foods that are not underlined and their consistency with cell composition.

Elixirs

Squeeze ½ vial of Essence directly under the tongue.

Squeeze ½ vial of Blood Rx directly under the tongue.

Squeeze ½ vial of Liver Rx directly under the tongue.

CHAPTER 15

Phase 2 Exercise Regimen

This phase of exercises will focus on generating, and then intensifying, lymph, oxygen and neural energy flow, particularly in the regions affecting your reproductive organs.

Aerobic vs. Anaerobic Exercising

At the core of aerobic and anaerobic exercising is the scientific fact that, to exercise, your body needs to break down sugar and then convert it to glycogen so that it can be utilized as energy or fuel. When your body has an adequate supply of oxygen for this process, we call it aerobic respiration. When there is not enough oxygen, like when an athlete runs hard or sprints at the end of a 5k, this is called anaerobic respiration. Aerobic, then, means "with oxygen", and anaerobic means "without oxygen".

When you exercise aerobically your muscles have enough oxygen to produce all the energy they need to perform. You breathe in, and your body efficiently uses all the oxygen it needs to power your muscles, and then you exhale. The waste products of aerobic respiration are carbon dioxide (CO2) and water. These byproducts are easily expelled through the simple act of breathing. This is why your breath is carbon dioxide rich and moist.

Anaerobic respiration happens when there is insufficient oxygen but nitrogen/ammonia present. In this instance, your muscles don't have enough oxygen to create the energy you are demanding from them (like carrying heavy furniture up stairs). When this happens muscles begin to break down essential sugars, but instead of producing CO2 and water, it produces free radicals and lactic acid (that burning-cramp sensation you feel in your shoulder muscles when you hold your arms out in front of you for too long). Unfortunately, lactic acid is harder to clear than water and CO2. Thus, lactic acid accumulates in your system, causing extreme fatigue.

During the Extermination phase you will be performing mostly aerobic exercises. This is of the utmost importance, as this phase is all about extracting and flushing out toxins, where the focus will be on healing your reproductive organs, tissues and muscles. When you exert excess energy on any other muscle, especially to the point of "feeling the burn", i.e., the muscle producing lactic acid, your body will naturally focus its repairing mechanisms to either heal or build that particular muscle, diminishing or distracting the focus away from healing your reproductive organs.

THE FOLLOWING SECTION IS DEDICATED TO YOUR SUCCESS THROUGH EXERCISE:

CHAPTER 16

Qi Gong

The Basics

Qi Gong is electric Health's number one choice in aerobic exercising. Qi Gong means "Life Energy Cultivation", and is the practice of aligning body, breath, and mind for health, meditation, and martial arts, i.e., your physiology and psychology. Your body is a complete system of inter and intra-dependent electro-magnetic energy fields (pathways). Each electro-magnetic field is respondent to your cells, glands and organs, through which your Qi (life energy) flows. The major electro-magnetic fields in your body are known as **meridians**. You have a total of 24 meridians; 12 standard meridians on the left side of your body, and 12 on the right.

12 Standard Meridians

The twelve standard meridians, also called Principal Meridians, are divided into **Yin** and **Yang** groups. Yin is an energy quality characterized as slow, soft, yielding, contracting, cold, wet, and passive; and is associated with water, earth, the moon, femininity, and nighttime. Yang, by contrast, is an energy quality that is characterized as fast, hard, solid, expanding, hot, dry, and aggressive; and is associated with fire, sky, the sun, masculinity and daytime.

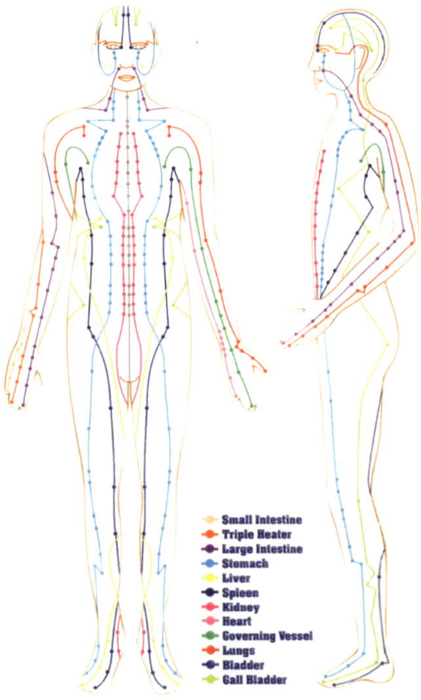

The Yin meridians of the arm are Lung, Heart, and Pericardium. The Yang meridians of the arm are Large Intestine, Small Intestine, and Triple Heater. The Yin Meridians of the leg are Spleen, Kidney, and Liver. The Yang meridians of the leg are Stomach, Bladder, and Gall Bladder. Qi Gong is the art of revitalizing, balancing yin and yang, and/or releasing flow of blocked or dysfunctional meridian pathways, with a combination of correct breathing techniques and precisely guided body movements.

Qi Gong Fibroid Elimination Exercises

Wu Ji Stance (Starting Position)

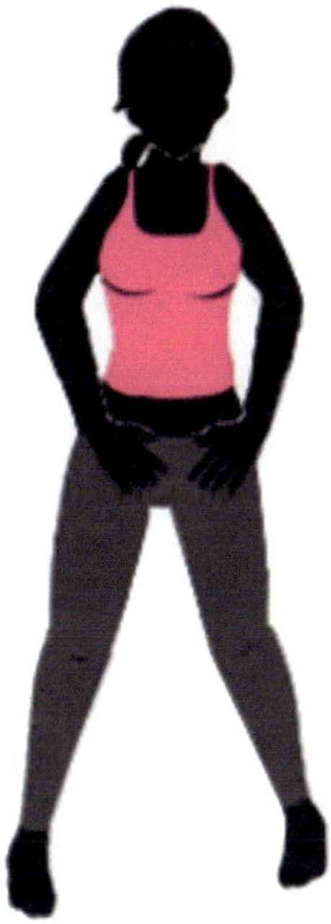

- Stand flat on your feet, with your toes pointing forward
- Your feet should be shoulder-width apart
- Bend your knees slightly as if you are holding a large beach ball between your legs
- Tighten your anus, only slightly, but keep your perineum sphincter relaxed
- Keep your arms at your sides, slightly opening your armpits, as if small balls have been placed under each of them
- This will result in your hands hanging relaxed just in front of you
- Pull in your stomach
- Close your eyes focusing your inner vision in the them in your headspace between
- Place the tip of your tongue on the gum line of your upper teeth

- Relax all parts of your body
- Breath softly and deeply through your nostrils, gently pushing the lower abdomen down on the "in breath", and pulling it up (not your chest) just as gently on the "out breath" (diaphragmatic breathing)
- This is the starting posture you will adopt in all the elimination Qi Gong exercises

The Wu Ji Stance is a powerful meditative standing position which, on its own, can be adopted at any time of the day to restore homeostasis (balance) to your entire body and mind

Gathering Yin (20 repetitions)

- Keeping your eyes open, stand in Wu Ji Stance (A) and begin breathing in for a count of 4
- Slowly swing your arms up and out, at your sides, within the 4 count in breath, through head to position (C) position (B) and above your
- Position (C) will end your in-breath
- Allow your body to fall forward freely (D) breathing out naturally without counting
- Touch the floor with your hands as if you are scooping the air (E), and return to (B) as you breath in slowly again for your next cycle

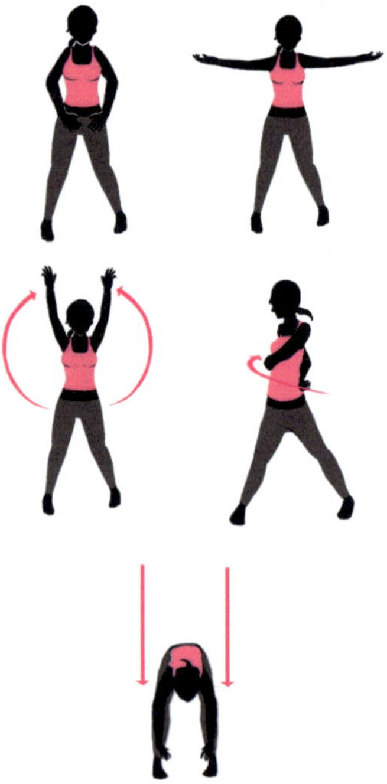

The gathering of yin serves to draw in, and then harness and internalize the earth's positive accumulated excess negative energies, whilst expelling the energies. It serves to process internal maintenance and flow of blood and energy throughout the various body systems, by removing restrictions and aiding in the reduction of internal growths, swellings and inflammation. It can also be performed at night before bed to ensure a good night's kip.

Turtle Breathing (12 repetitions)

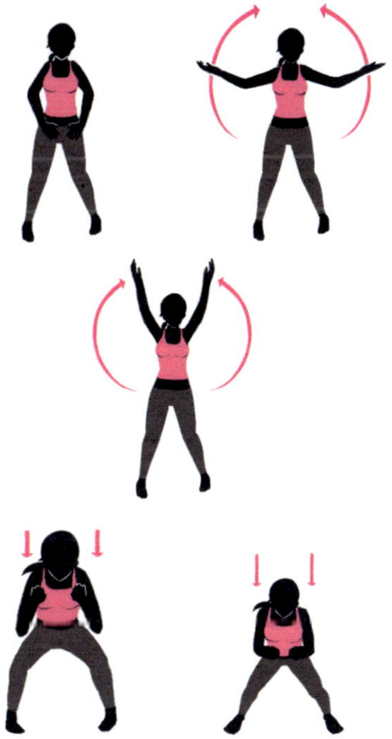

- Stand in Wu Ji Stance (A). On the count of 1 of the 4 count in-breath, slowly swing your arms up and out to the side (palms up)
- Through the counts 2 and 3 continue slowly raising the arms through (B)
- Your arm movement ends above your head at (C) ending your in-breath
- As you breathe out for 4 counts lower your body to a squatting position (D) hands making a fist. Keep your back straight and do not lean forward.
- Leaning forward (E) release your fists and lower your hands, with palms facing you. Breathe in quickly and gently, contracting and releasing your perineum gently 8 times (the perineum is the muscle that you contract to stop your urine in midstream or to hold your urine)
- At the end of your contractions begin breathing in as you raise your body up through position (B), beginning a new cycle repetition

As suggested by its name, turtle breathing is an exercise which provides longevity to its host, by tonifying and strengthening those organs, namely the liver, kidneys, uterus, and perineum, which, functioning in their respective optimal capacities, maintain health, youth and deter aging.

"Yu" Bladder Stasis Deep Healing (up to 50 repetitions)

- You don't need to stand in Wu Ji Stance. Spread legs wider than shoulder width.
- Make a diamond shape with your hands, placing your touching thumbs over your navel, and your finger tips just above your genital area (A)
- Breathe in for a count of 4, expanding the diaphragm
- Chant "Yu" as you breath out for a count of 4, turning your body completely to the right without moving your feet (B)
- Breathe in for a count of 4 as you turn towards position (C)
- Chant "Yu" as you breathe out for a count of 4, turning your body completely to the left without moving your feet (D)
- Breathe in for a count of 4 as you return to position (A)

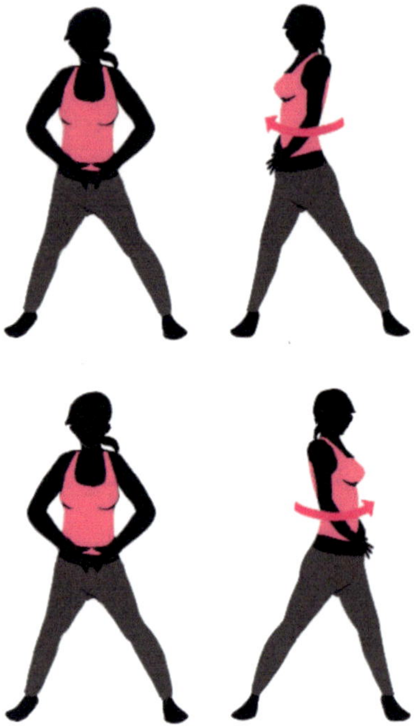

The bladder stasis deep healing exercise is very powerful. It helps to maintain the optimal health of male and female reproductive organs. It is highly reputed to assist in disintegrating tumors of both the prostate and ovaries. This is one of the key elements of our fibroid elimination process.

"Gong" Spleen Stasis Deep Healing (up to 50 repetitions)

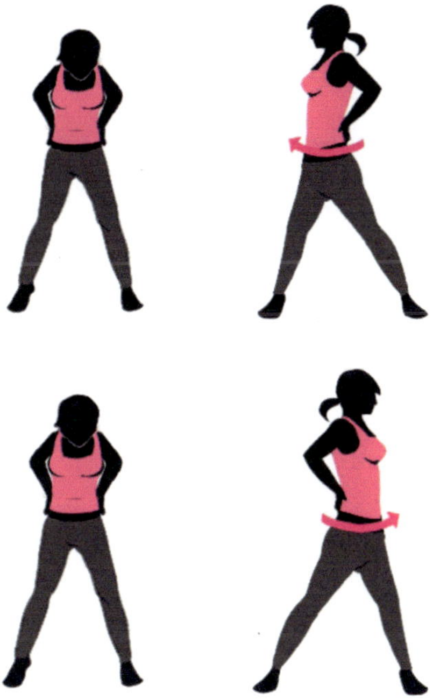

- You don't need to stand in Wu Ji Stance. Spread legs wider than shoulder width, looking down at the floor, about 3 feet in front of you
- Place your hands on the sides of your lower back (A) and breathe in for a count of 4
- Chant "Gong" as you breath out for a count of 4, turning your body completely to the right, and pivoting your left foot for balance (B)
- Breathe in for a count of 4 as you turn towards position (C)
- Chant "Gong" as you breath out for a count of 4, turning your body completely to the left, and pivoting your right foot for balance (D)
- Breathe in for a count of 4 as you return to position (A)

The spleen stasis deep healing exercise is paramount in relieving painful menses, endometriosis and all other uterine growth disorders. Use with caution if your menstrual flow is extremely heavy.

CHAPTER 17

Phase 2 Exercise Calendar

	DAYS 1, 8, 15	DAYS 2, 9, 16	DAYS 3, 10, 17	DAYS 4, 11, 18	DAYS 5, 12, 19	DAYS 6, 13, 20	DAYS 7, 14, 21
7AM	GATHER YIN TURTLE BREATH YU BLAD-DER	GATHER YIN TURTLE BREATH GONG SPLEEN	GATHER YIN TURTLE BREATH YU BLAD-DER	GATHER YIN TURTLE BREATH GONG SPLEEN	GATHER YIN TURTLE BREATH YU BLAD-DER	GATHER YIN TURTLE BREATH GONG SPLEEN	GATHER YIN TURTLE BREATH YU BLAD-DER
1PM	SQUATS	SQUATS	SQUATS	SQUATS	SQUATS	SQUATS	SQUATS
8PM	GATHER YIN TURTLE BREATH YU BLAD-DER	GATHER YIN TURTLE BREATH GONG SPLEEN	GATHER YIN TURTLE BREATH YU BLAD-DER	GATHER YIN TURTLE BREATH GONG SPLEEN	GATHER YIN TURTLE BREATH YU BLAD-DER	GATHER YIN TURTLE BREATH GONG SPLEEN	GATHER YIN TURTLE BREATH GONG SPLEEN

Detox, Detox, Detox!

The main purpose of this phase is to deprive, and thus starve, your fibroids of their food supply without cutting off the blood supply and oxygen to your uterus. We have already identified and proven that the true, main culprit behind your condition is estrogen, in its many forms. Strict implementation and execution of the Estrogen Fast and the eHealth Lifestyle Food List, respectively, are therefore absolutely mandatory.

The eHealth Lifestyle Food List is fortified with minerals that are aromatase and estrogen inhibitors. The Essence™ elixir is added to your herbal supplements in this phase. This is the fibroid executioner – imagine the Blood Rx™ and Liver Rx™ as the executioner's two henchmen who disable, and then restrain your microscopic assailants. Now, visualize the food that you will be eating over the next

21 days as either reinforcements to the executioner or, adversely, reinforcement agents to your fibroids. It is that plain and simple, black and white, on or off…the choice is yours.

Ready…Steady…GO, GO, GO!

Daily and regular bowel movements are essential to your fibroid extermination. Imagine the garbage at your house: if you neglect to take it out, it will pile up, start smelling pretty obnoxious, attract all types of vermin, and quickly become a major blight upon your neighborhood. During your fibroid extermination phase your body is taking out its garbage by eliminating the mass array of toxins, mainly through the bowels. Having daily and regular bowel movements will ensure that your toxins are not maintained, re-assimilated or re-absorbed back into your system. The frequency of your bowel movements will increase while going through the extermination phase. If for some reason you experience constipation, follow this mini-guide to resolve your blockage:

- Hydrate, Hydrate, Hydrate: Increase your water intake so that you use the bathroom approximately once every hour.

- Increase the Fiber: Eat more green leafy vegetables, black cherries, figs, lukewarm lemon water, watermelons, and green vegetable smoothies.

- Dance & Prance: Do some movement and exercise. Qi Gong is excellent for this, or simply walk!

- Use The Sweeper™: Electric pHood's very powerful elixir formulated specifically to regenerate and enhance digestive organs and the alimentary tract, to ensure foods are being properly digested, and all nutrients are being fully absorbed.

Cold & Flu-like Symptoms

You will be eradicating not only the estrogen dominant substances from your body, but also the parasites that have joined the party over years of bad habits, and that have become permanent residents in your body's systems and organs. Parasites are bacteria, fungi, viruses, and yeast spores. They have developed a symbiotic relationship with your cells and are not going to leave without a fight!!!

The ensuing fight or conflict, which may feel like a viral illness, will be acute but the severity or intensity depends totally upon the severity of your infestation(s) – from mild sweats and sniffles, to headaches, nausea, diarrhea and shivers, and everything in between.

Skin Rashes & Eczema Outbreaks

The largest organ through which your body discharges poisons and parasites is the intestines. Other main organs of excretion are the liver, the kidneys and the lungs (via the respiratory system). Your skin is also a main organ of excretion. Often, when your body is dysfunctional, some of these organs, namely, the intestines, kidneys and lungs, perform their respective poison excretion duties rather poorly, and your skin is forced to become a major organ of excretion. If this is the case, it will explain the sudden eruptions of skin surface rashes and eczema. Though you cannot detect it, the poisons in your body are rapidly discharged through your skin eruptions, so you should not fret or treat these outbreaks as villainous. These outbreaks will only be temporary as the combination of your new diet, the elixirs and the exercise regimen will restore your other excretion organs to optimum functionality.

Those Dreaded Cravings

The relationship between you and the parasites that have infested your body is a chemical one. They have infiltrated your bloodstream, penetrated your lymphatic system, and breached your central nervous system. In their colonial efforts, they have assimilated a symbiotic influence, of mesmeric proportions, over both your physiological and psychological behavior, by mimicking hormones that, in turn, manifest as physical and mental cravings. What you may believe are "legitimate" compulsions, during this phase of "poison deprivation", are, in actuality, the desperate chemical attempts of these parasites to save themselves from certain death. We strongly discourage snacking during this phase. Snacking is the precursor, initiator and mother of all bad eating habits. This will be, without a doubt, your most trying times, but you must execute will power, inner strength and determination, to see it through. Just remember why you're doing this, and always focus on your end game. If you absolutely must snack, fruits and/or veggie juices (smoothies) from our recipes will compensate greatly for your cravings.

CHAPTER 18

Good Old H2O

One of the greatest impediments of patients achieving a successful detox, and the fundamental flaw observed with those same patients' lifestyles, often rest in their mis-educated choices when it comes to drinking water. This section is therefore dedicated to dispelling the conjecture and myths surrounding this, somewhat, controversial topic, and to shed a beacon of light that will guide you on the correct path, so that you will never partake in any unnecessary or counterproductive water consumption.

- Buying bottled water can be a deceptive and dangerous practice, especially if you don't have the necessary tools to test its alkalinity. Most bottled waters on the market, claiming to be spring or artesian water, are nothing more than bulk tap water that has been "purified" (we hope) and re-bottled for sale. Bulk water is water that has lost its natural structure and is usually recycled, chemically infused, urbanized water. The bulk water molecule is often too large to penetrate the human cell membrane so does not hydrate the cell. At best it only performs a flushing effect as it swiftly runs through the body, dragging out only a few impurities in its wake. The cell will thus remain dehydrated and deoxygenated, and toxins will remain untroubled within the cell. Rapid cellular degeneration will ensue and disease is inevitable.

- Contrary to popular belief, it is possible to drink too much alkaline water. Whilst we encourage our patients to down plenty of water during and after any detox, we must warn that the body and brain requires a certain amount of structural acidity to maintain specific tissues, organs and glands, and to perform major systemic functions. If the body is overwhelmed with alkalinity, its acid-alkaline homeostasis is polarized, which will diminish its ability to properly carry out its many functions, which will cause major dysfunction and illnesses.

- Ionized water is not good for you, especially in the long-run. Natural water is alkaline due to its mineral content. The natural molecular structure for water contains both positive and negative charges. Some minerals attach or bond to the slightly positively charged (hydrogen) ions and

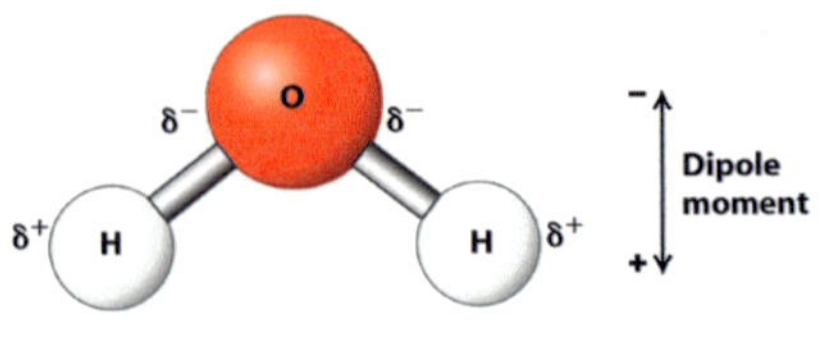

the rest bond to the negatively charged (oxygen) ions. This is called **structured water**. Man-made machines have made it possible to ionize (or de- structure) the water, meaning the water is separated into its two distinct (positive or negative) charges. This is called de-natured water. We drink the negatively charged (alkaline) portion, and we either discard the positively charged (acidic) portion, or use it for disinfecting/cleaning purposes. De-natured (hybrid) water lacks its hydrogen wholeness and is effectively deficient of half its minerals. Further, most people who own ionizing machines use tap water, which is already devoid of essential minerals, and also containing toxins, such as heavy metals, arsenic, etc. The ionizer synthetically charges the water and then separates it into its two distinct polarities without filtering out the toxins. The human body is fooled into believing the water contains alkaline minerals, which are the necessary nutrients, but it cannot and does not draw any from the water. Instead the hybrid water draws the minerals from the body in an attempt to become structured again, and systematically and eventually depletes the body of its essential minerals.

- Distilled water can be analogized as a reverse Jekyll and Hyde. In its pure form it is an aggressive beast that, when ingested, immediately seeks to regain its minerals (lost in the distillation process) by sucking them out of the cells, tissues, organs, or bones. By simply adding trace minerals or a few drops of wild chlorophyll to it before drinking, distilled water becomes your anatomical best friend, full of life and devoid of all harmful impurities. Distilled water can be purchased at extremely cheap prices at your local supermarket. An absolute win-win situation.

- The BEST source for structured water is in wild or organic fruits, mountain streams, artesian wells, or natural springs.

- Unless you live in the Swiss Alps, or some other lucky place in Scandinavia, LEAVE TAP WATER ALONE!!!

- While detoxing, perform the following simple task to calculate the general amount of water to drink daily, depending upon your physical constitution:

    - Find out your weight in pounds

- Divide by 2
- Substitute the figure amount in pounds to the same figure in ounces
- Divide that amount by 8
- The result is the amount of 8oz glasses of water you should drink daily

- It is important to note that this is just a "general" guide to the amount of water that you should drink daily. Your physical constitution, and its overall polarity, will ultimately be the deciding factor of the "best" amount of water for you consume each day. Positively charged individuals can drink and thrive off large amounts of water, whereas negatively charged individuals must limit their water intake. If you experience hypersensitivity to cold, feel bloated, and feel fatigued while executing the above formula, discard it and decrease your amount of water intake immediately. It means that your body is negatively charged, and too much water will result in adverse effects on your body and wellbeing.

CHAPTER 19

Phase 3: Regeneration

If you have completed the extermination phase (CONGRATULATIONS) your fibroids should at least have diminished significantly and/or be almost completely gone. Your other "old and unwanted baggage" that will have suffered the same fate includes, but is not limited to, fat and excess weight. Your energy levels, including your libido, should be noticeably increasing each day, and you should appear and feel much younger.

There are two main purposes of this phase:

- To regenerate, develop, tone and sustain your muscle tissue that may have been collaterally lost during extermination.

- To regenerate, develop, tone and sustain essential reproductive muscle tissue that, due to neglect, may have atrophied over the course of your adult life.

Muscle Tissue

There are 3 types of muscle tissue:

- Skeletal or striated muscles, those that move the skeleton (also called voluntary muscle).

- Cardiac muscle, which makes up most of the heart wall (also an involuntary muscle).

- Smooth muscles (also called involuntary muscle), such as the muscles contained in the stomach and other internal organs.

Your focus in this phase will be on the striated and smooth muscles. Cardiac muscle toning will be omitted, as the health of your heart, hopefully, is not a concern. Striated or skeletal muscles are the muscles that we traditionally "work out" to either build or tone. Work outs for smooth muscles, which include your reproductive organs, are seldom advertised or, for that matter, taught, so most people don't even know that they exist. We will be implementing a combination of aerobic and anaerobic exercises, but first…

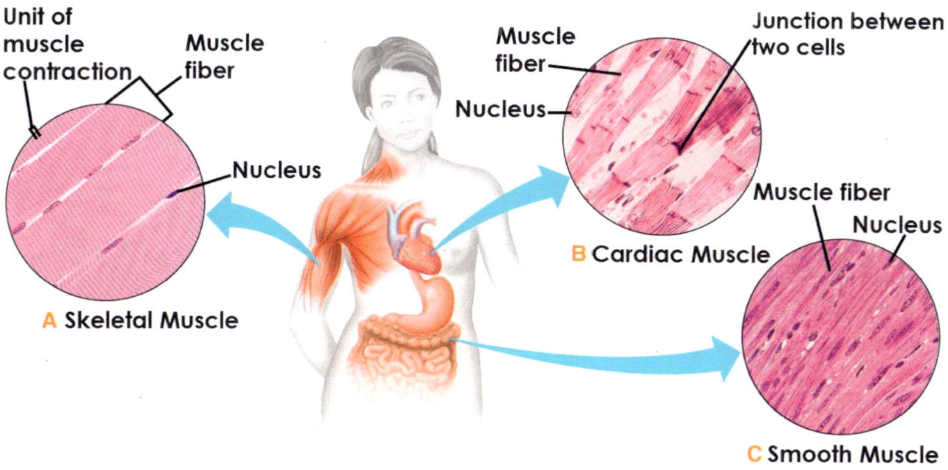
Unit of muscle contraction
Muscle fiber
Nucleus
A Skeletal Muscle
Muscle fiber
Nucleus
Junction between two cells
B Cardiac Muscle
Muscle fiber
Nucleus
C Smooth Muscle

CHAPTER 20

The Regeneration Diet (Class C)

9 DAYS (and beyond)

Eat 3 meals a day, including the specific eHealth Recipe Smoothie. Use ONLY foods selected from the electric Health Lifestyle Food List.

As with Phase 2, there are no alternatives. Carefully plan your daily meals, for at least the next 9 days. After the 9 days are complete, you may venture, to other healthy, Class C recipes outside the realms of electric Health, but DO NOT return to any Class Diet below C.

Your Phase 3 Daily Diet Plan

8am – 11am	12pm – 3pm	5pm – 7pm	9pm – 10pm
Breakfast	**Lunch**	**Dinner**	**Night Cap**
Fruit Smoothie	Main Meal	Grain-Enhanced Dinner	Fruits or Smoothie
+ **Elixirs**	+ **Elixirs**	+ **Elixirs**	

Breakfast

Lemon & Breakfast Recipe

Start your day with a fresh organic lemon, squeezing the juice directly under your tongue, followed by eating the whole pulp. This will infuse essential negatively charged ions directly into your bloodstream. This is done prior to your first daily exercise regimen. After your workout, be sure to blend a fresh smoothie with your own choice of ingredients from the electric Health Eat List.

Elixirs

Squeeze ½ vial of Essence directly under the tongue.

Squeeze ½ vial of Blood Rx directly under the tongue.

Squeeze ½ vial of Liver Rx directly under the tongue.

Lunch

eHealth Main Meal Recipe

This is your heaviest meal of the day. Select your meal from the eHealth Main Meal Recipe list. Again, this is your main and most essential meal. The timing is directly in tune with your natural appropriation cycle, so that it is fully digested well before the initiation of the assimilation cycle. This is the most effective time to eat dark green leafy vegetables, and seeds, such as quinoa, for your protein. It is important for us to stress that this is not a weight loss diet, even though, during this phase, you are guaranteed to lose weight. To this end, we strongly recommend that 50% of your daily intake be of the seeds in our list. Seeds contain the essential amino and carboxylic acids to develop and maintain muscle mass, strength and vitality.

Elixirs

Squeeze ½ vial of Essence directly under the tongue.

Squeeze ½ vial of Blood Rx directly under the tongue.

Squeeze ½ vial of Liver Rx directly under the tongue.

Dinner

electric Health Seed-Enhanced Dinner Recipe

Prepare a seed-based meal including a fruit salad. It is imperative that these meals contain super seeds, especially hemp seeds and quinoa, and plenty of green leafy vegetables, such as black kale.

Elixirs

Squeeze ½ vial of Essence directly under the tongue. Squeeze ½ vial of Blood Rx directly under the tongue.

Squeeze ½ vial of Liver Rx directly under the tongue.

CHAPTER 21

Phase 3 Exercise Regimen

As stated previously, this phase of exercises will focus on building and toning both, skeletal muscle tissue that may have decreased during the extermination phase, and the reproductive and contributing smooth muscle tissue that may have atrophied over the course of your adult life, by implementing a combination of aerobic and anaerobic resistance exercises. When performing anaerobic exercises, take regular sips of organic fruit juice to supply antioxidants to your muscles (we highly recommend black/purple grape juice and/or freshly squeezed lemon juice). This neutralizes the lactic acid and, thus, prevents build up.

Qi Gong Tonification Exercises

Gathering Yang (20 breath-cycle repetitions)

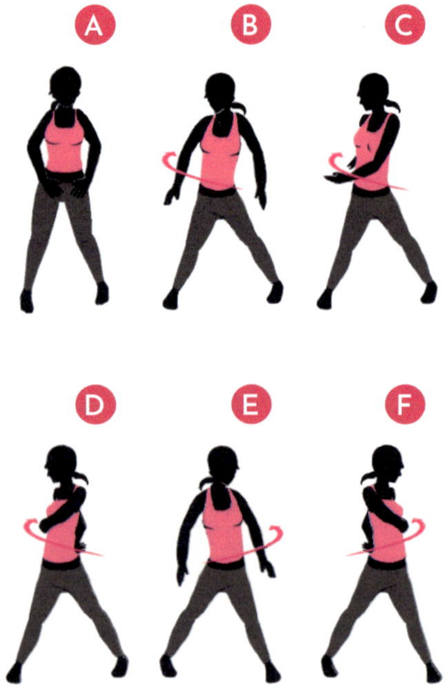

- Keeping your eyes open, stand in Wu Ji Stance (A) with your legs slightly wider apart than usual
- Lower your arms to your sides and breathe in for a count of 4, begin swinging your body to your right at a brisk pace, letting your arms follow loosely through (B), (C), and (D)
- At your extreme right, quickly begin swinging your body at the same pace, through (E), and (F), all the way to your extreme left
- Repeat motions (B) to (F) through your 4 count in-breath, and then repeat the same motions through your out- breath, to complete one breath-cycle
- Immediately start the next breath-cycle repetition to the desired amount.

Kidney Tonification (20 repetitions per side)

- Stand with feet slightly wider apart than Wu Ji Stance
- Place your right palm behind your back and on your left kidney
- Begin breathing in for a count of 4, while extending your left hand up and across your body to your right side through (A) and ending with your arm extended at shoulder height (B) ending the in-breath
- Begin breathing out for a count of 4, leaning back towards your left, moving and keeping your left height through position (C) arm at shoulder
- As your left hand passes your face, begin to lower your body, in a circular motion, toward the left side floor, maintaining the distance between your hand and face, while keeping your eyes affixed to your hand (D), ending the out-breath when you are fully inclined to the side
- Breathe in for 4 as you scoop air from the floor, still maintaining a circular motion, raising back up to your right (E)
- Complete your circular motion and in-breath with your arm fully extended and at shoulder length (F)

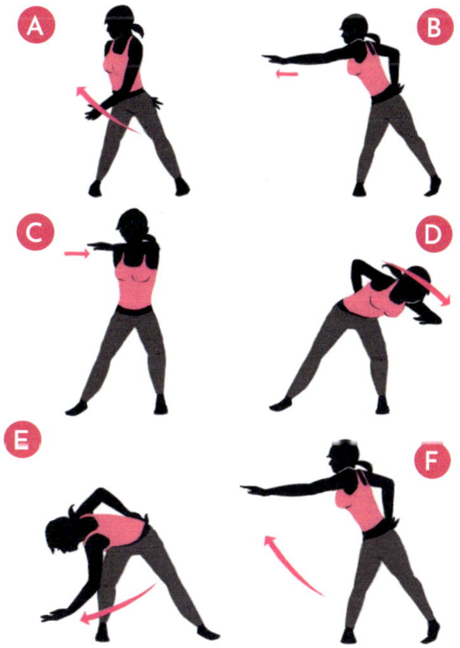

- Continue repetitions to your desired goal and then switch arms and direction to exercise the right kidney

The daily practice of the kidney tonification exercise, coupled with a correct diet, will drastically inhibit the aging process which, itself, is an illness. The kidney tonification sequence will also eliminate the following conditions:

- Poor recuperation from rest (adrenal insufficiency)
- Premature graying (graying hair is a sign of kidney dysfunction)
- Premature balding (balding is an illness)
- Osteoporosis and other skeletal issues
- Tooth decay
- Anemia
- Infertility
- Hormonal imbalances/deficiencies
- Senility
- Weakness of legs
- Lower back pains

Lung Tonification (40 repetitions)

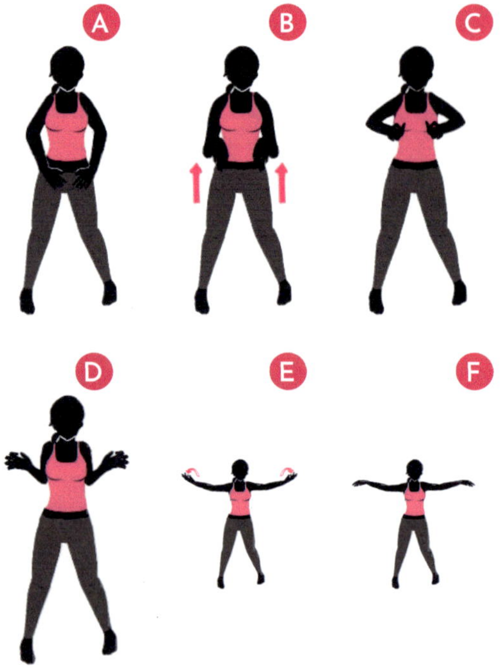

Stand in Wu Ji Stance and close your eyes

As you begin the 4-count in-breath, raise your hands front of you to chest height (A)

Continue the in-breath as you turn your palms upwards through (B) and end the in-breath at (C), palms up

Begin the 4-count out-breath as you open your arms an move them backwards to align with your body, pal facing upwards (D)

End the out-breath by rotating your hands so they end u palms facing down (E)

Breathe in for 4 counts as you move your arms upwards returning them stretched to front and center of your chest palms down (F). Repeat (B) thru (F) for desired repetitions

Liver Tonification (25 repetitions each side)

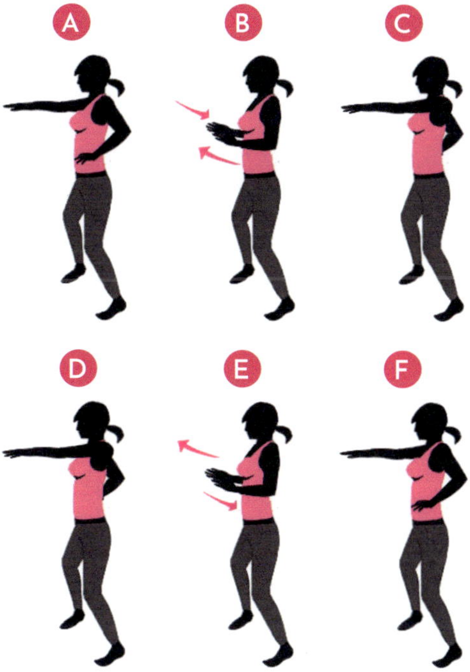

- Stand in position (A) with your right arm extended out in front of you at 90°, left arm tucked to your side and slightly raised
- Breathe in for a count of 4, pulling your right arm back and pushing your left arm forward, almost touching hands as they pass each other midway (B)
- End the in-breath at position (C), with extended in front of you at 90°
- Begin breathing out at position (D) your left arm full
- Breathe out for a count of 4, pulling your left arm back and pushing your right arm forward, again almost touching hands as they pass each other midway (E)
- End the out-breath at position (F), with your right arm fully extended in front of you at 90°
- Repeat positions (B) thru (F) for 25 breathing cycles, then perform another 25 repetitions, this time starting by pulling the left hand back first at the in-breath.

CHAPTER 22

eHealth Regeneration Exercises

Alternating Lateral Lunge: 5 repetitions x 3 sets (add 2 reps per day)

- Holding a pair of 10 lb dumbbells at your sides, stand in position A.
- Step out to the left with your left leg; bend your knee and sit back to lower into a side lunge, keeping your back flat as you lower the right dumbbell to the inside of the left foot into position B.
- Press through the left foot to return to start. That completes 1 repetition.
- Repeat on the other side. Continue alternating for appropriate reps on each side.

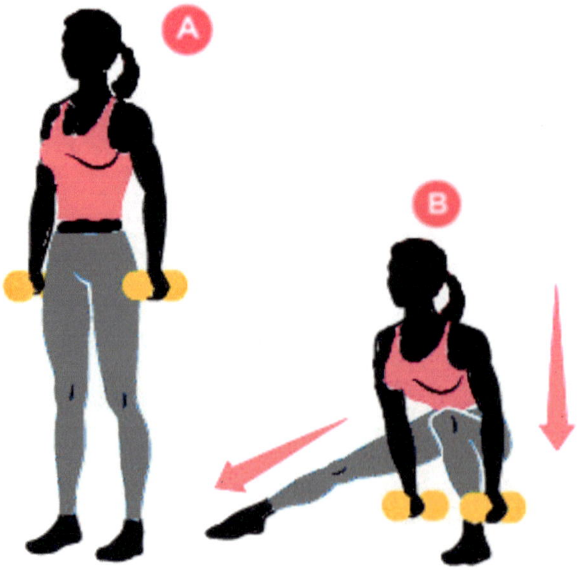

Dumbbell Curl Squat Press: 7 repetitions x 3 sets (add 2 reps per day)

- A: Start with your feet shoulder width apart and the 10 lb weights in each hand on the side of your body standing straight up.
- B: Slowly sit down into a squat position while curling the dumbbells to your shoulders.
- C: Slowly stand back up, pressing the weight over your head with your palms facing inward.
- Bring the weight back down to your waste. This completes one repetition.

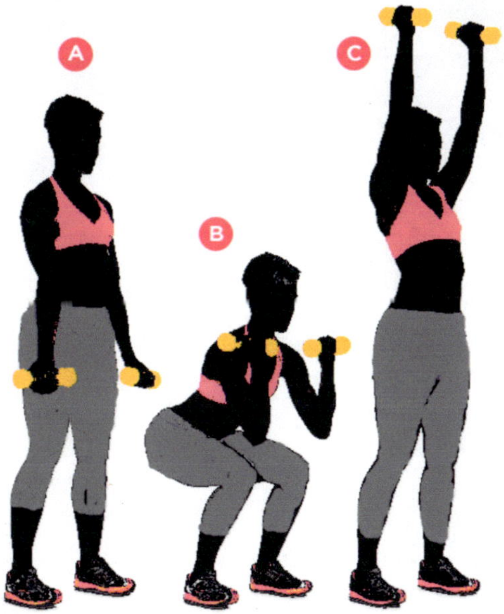

Front Kick: 7 repetitions x 3 sets each leg (add 2 reps per day)

- Stand with your legs slightly apart, and raise your fists like you're protecting your face.
- Bring your right knee up to position A.
- Quickly extend your raised leg out in front of you to position B and return to position A.
- Repeat 5 times, and then switch legs.

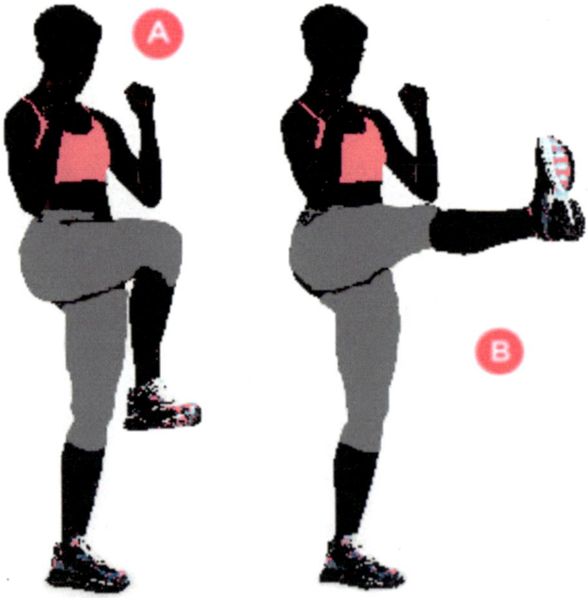

Golf Squat: 7 repetitions x 3 sets (add 2 reps per day)

- Stand with your feet more than hip-width apart, holding a 15 lb dumbbell with both hands in front of your body.
- Keeping your chest upright, bend your knees to lower into a squat (A).
- As you stand, rotate your torso to the left while raising the dumbbell over your shoulder (like you're swinging a golf club) (B).
- Return to start; repeat, rotating to the right side. That's one rep

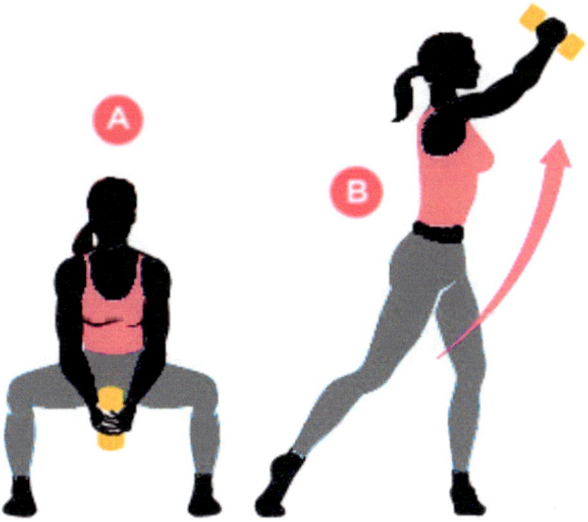

Large Butterfly Sit-ups: 15 repetitions x 3 sets (add 2 reps per day)

- Lie on your back while placing both of your legs in the frog position A, by putting the bottom of both your feet together.
- Sit up keeping your back straight and still with your arms stretched in front of you to reach the tip of your toes (B).
- If you want to make the movement more difficult, you can place your hands on your chest.
- Exhale and slowly turn back to the first position.

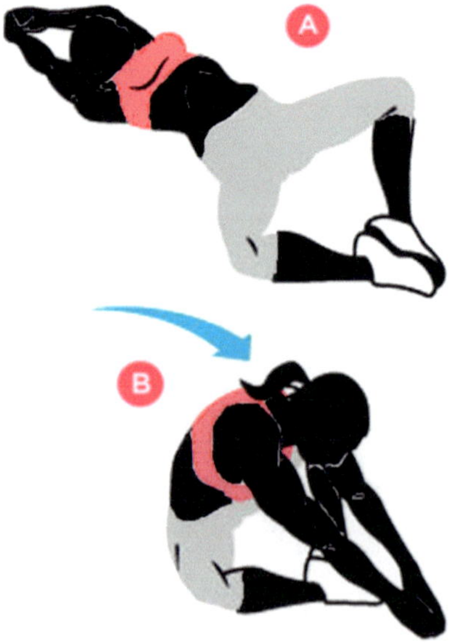

Lateral Leg Lift: 15 repetitions x 3 sets each leg (add 2 reps per day)

- With your hands on your hips and your feet hip-width apart, bend your knees to lower into a squat (A).
- Pause, then stand and lift your right leg out to the side as high as you can (B).
- Return to start. That's one rep.
- Repeat with the left leg, and continue alternating until you've done your complete set of reps on each side.

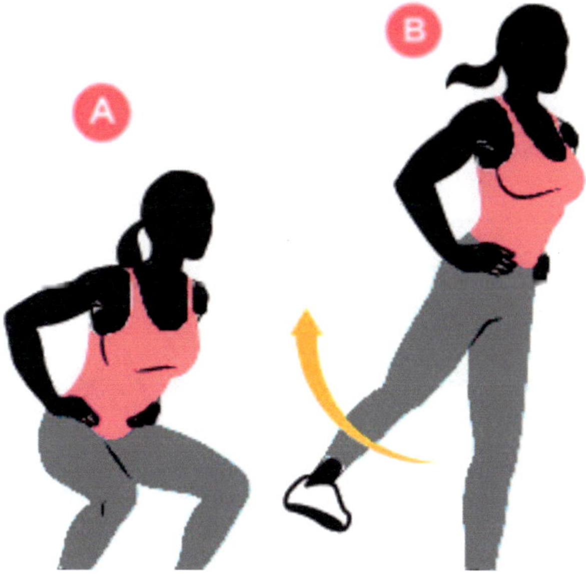

Oblique Crunch: 15 repetitions x 3 sets each side (add 2 reps per day)

- Lie flat on your back and bend your knees.
- Before crunching, turn your legs at the hips, all the way until the legs are both resting on the ground to one side (A).
- Flatten your lower back against the ground and curl upward, with your hands placed behind the head (B). It is more beneficial to hold the crunch position for a two count at the height of the curl.
- After performing your set number of Oblique Crunches on one side, twist your legs to the other side and perform the same number of crunches.

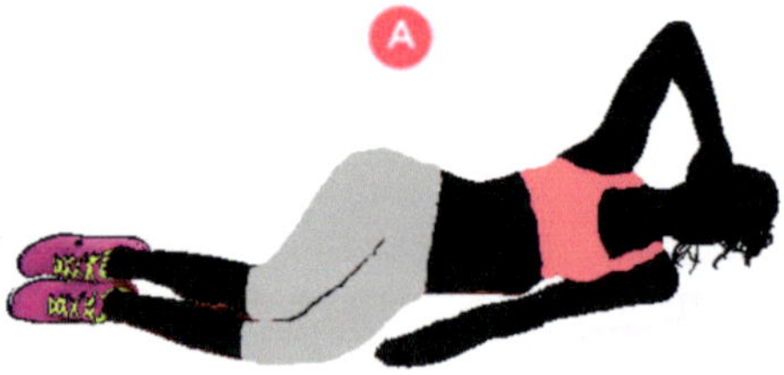

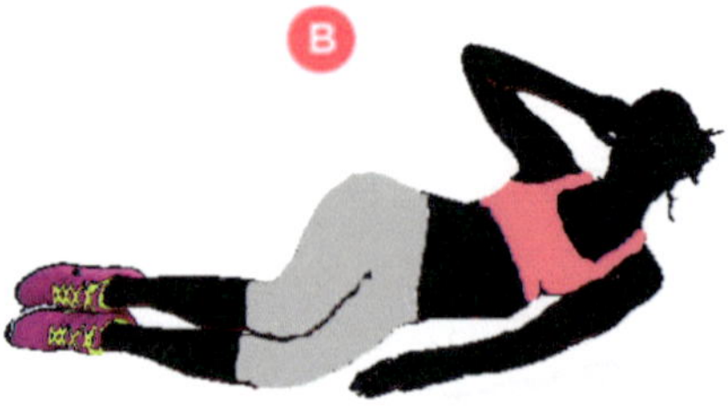

Oblique V-Up: 15 repetitions x 3 sets each side (add 2 reps per day)

- Lie on your left side, legs angled 30 degrees from your hips.
- Rest your left arm on the floor and put your right hand behind your head (A).
- Lift your straight legs off the floor, bringing your torso toward your legs (B).
- Slowly return to start. That's one rep. Do designated reps on each side.

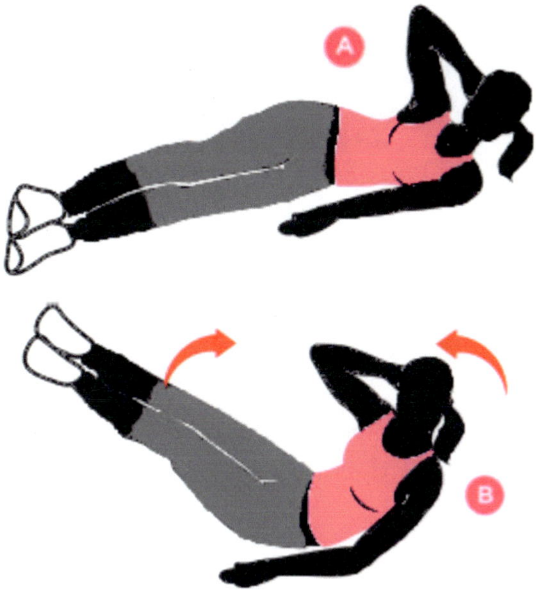

Rock 'n' Raise: 15 repetitions x 3 sets (add 2 reps per day)

- Lie on your back with your arms at your sides, your knees pointed outward, and the soles of your feet touching (A).
- Staying in this pose, slowly raise your legs until your toes are pointed toward the ceiling and your hips are slightly off the floor (B).
- Slowly return to start. That's one rep. Repeat to complete your designated amount.

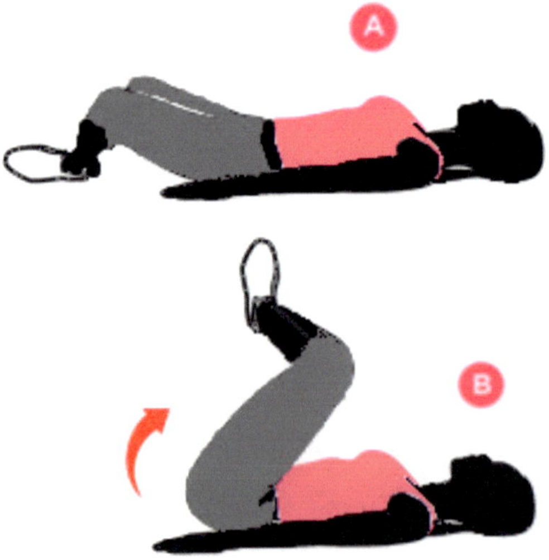

Side Leg Raise: 15 repetitions x 1 set each side

- Lie on your left side, rest your head on your left arm, and place your right hand on the floor in front of your chest (A).
- Your legs should be straight with your right leg on top of your left leg.
- Without moving any other part of your body, slowly raise your right leg as high as you can (B).
- Hold for 10 seconds, then return to the starting position. That's one rep. Do designated reps on each side.

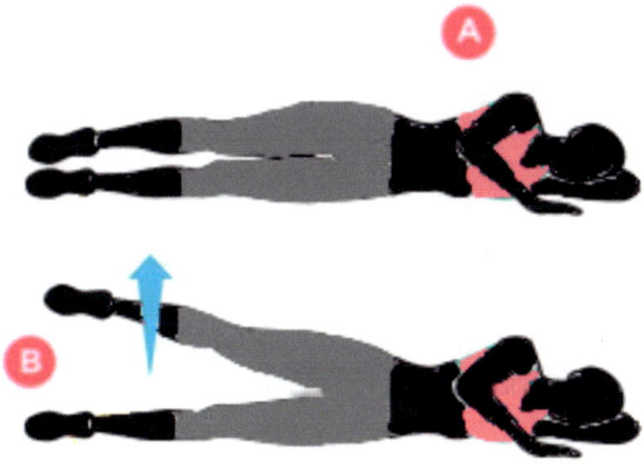

Side Scissor Kicks: 10 repetitions x 1 set each side

- Lie on your right side, all straight, propped up on one elbow.
- Lift your left leg slowly, keeping both legs straight (A). Hold it in the air for 10 seconds.
- Keeping your left leg in its same position, slowly raise your right leg until the insides of your feet touch (B). Hold this position for 10 seconds.
- Slowly lower your left leg back to its starting position. This is one rep.
- Raise right leg to repeat position B for the same count. Do designated reps on each side.

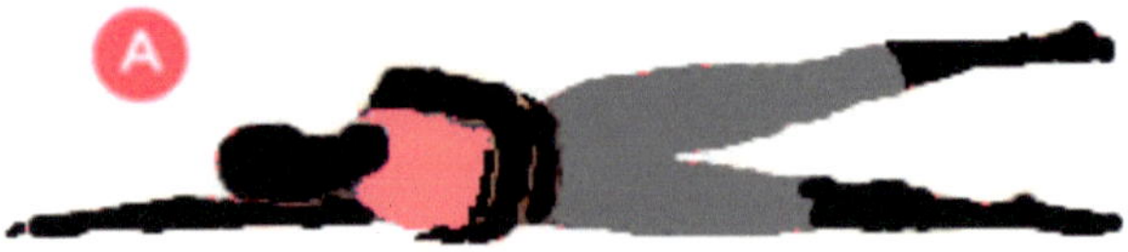

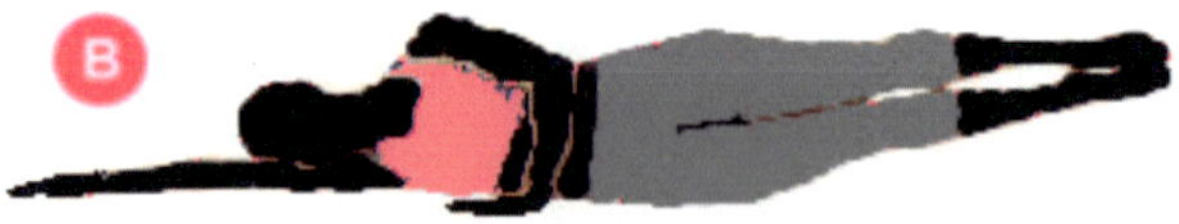

Simple Bridge: 15 repetitions x 1 set (add 2 reps per day)

- Lay flat on your back with your arms flat at your sides.
- Lift your hips into the air, keeping your arms flat but bending your knees.
- Hold the position at least 15 to 20 seconds, longer if you can.
- Slowly lower your hips back to position A. This is one rep. Repeat to your designated amount.

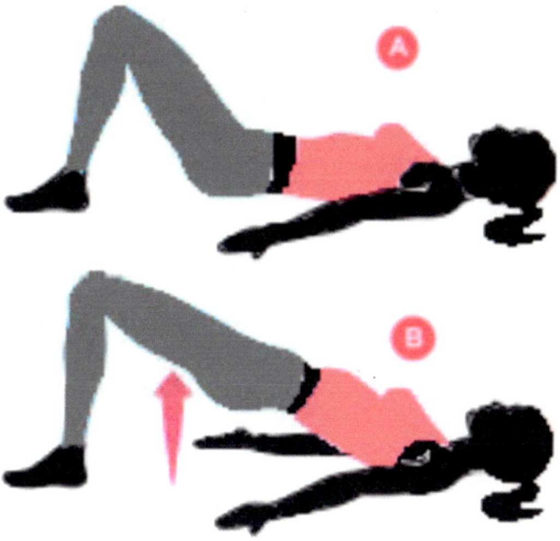

Single-Leg Hip Raise: 15 repetitions x 1 set

- Lie face-up on the floor with your left knee bent and your right leg straight. Raise your right leg until it's in line with your left thigh. (A)
- Push your hips upward, keeping your right leg elevated. (B)
- Hold for 10 seconds, and then slowly lower your body and leg back to the start position.
- Complete the prescribed number of repetitions with your left leg, then switch and do the same number with your right leg.

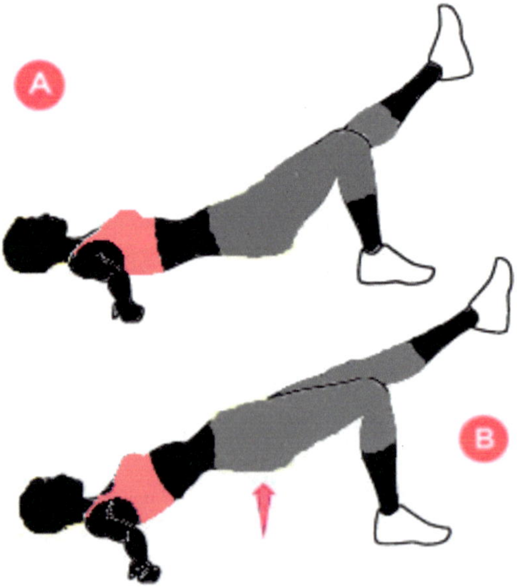

Squat Jumps: 15 repetitions x 3 sets (add 2 reps per day)

- A: Stand with your feet hip-width apart, toes forward; lightly touch your fingers behind your ears and extend your elbows to the sides.
- B: Slowly Bend your knees sitting into a squat, keeping your arms in their same position
- C: Maintaining your arm positions, explosively jump as high as you can.
- Landing softly on the balls of your feet, immediately lower into your next squat repetition.

It is imperative that the dumbbell(s) which you choose to use in the aforementioned exercises, actually offer resistance. Do not be afraid of increasing the weight. Resistance training has been proven to reduce the risk of osteoporosis. If you don't have sufficient weights equipment or the desired floor space at your home, we strongly recommend (in fact we insist) that you make the effort to join your local gym to proficiently perform the eHealth regeneration exercises detailed above.

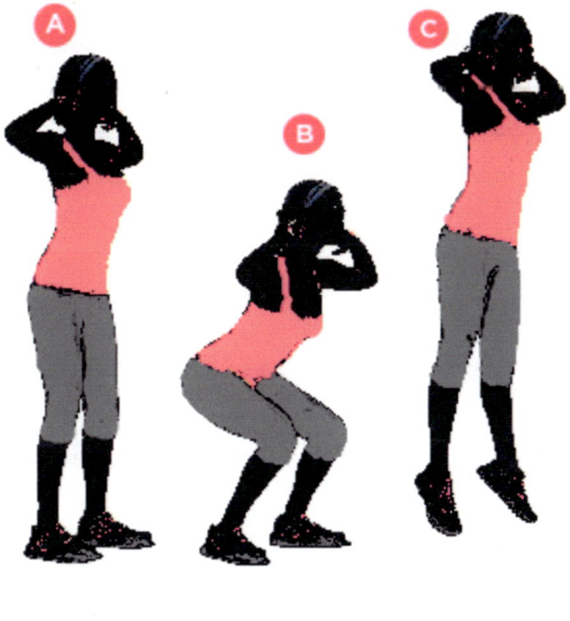

PHASE 3 DAYTIME EXERCISE CALENDAR

	EXERCISE I	EXERCISE II	EXERCISE III	EXERCISE IV	EXERCISE V	EXERCISE VI
DAY 1	GATHER YANG	KIDNEY TONIFICATION	LARGE BUTTERFLY SIT-UPS	ROCK AND RAISE	SIMPLE BRIDGE	LATERAL LEG LIFT
DAY 2	GATHER YANG	LIVER TONIFICATION	SQUAT JUMPS	FRONT KICKS	OBLIQUE V-UPS	SINGLE-LEG HIP RAISE
DAY 3	GATHER YANG	LUNGS TONIFICATION	DUMBBELL CURL SQUAT PRESS	ALTERNATING LATERAL LUNGE	GOLF SQUAT	SIDE LEG RAISE
DAY 4	GATHER YANG	KIDNEY TONIFICATION	LARGE BUTTERFLY SIT-UPS	ROCK AND RAISE	SIMPLE BRIDGE	LATERAL LEG LIFT
DAY 5	GATHER YANG	LIVER TONIFICATION	SQUAT JUMPS	FRONT KICKS	OBLIQUE CRUNCHES	SINGLE-LEG HIP RAISE
DAY 6	GATHER YANG	LUNGS TONIFICATION	DUMBBELL CURL SQUAT	ALTERNATING LATERAL LUNGE	GOLF SQUAT	SIDE SCISSOR KICKS
DAY 7	GATHER YANG	KIDNEY TONIFICATION	LARGE BUTTERFLY SIT-UPS	ROCK AND RAISE	SIMPLE BRIDGE	LATERAL LEG LIFT
DAY 8	GATHER YANG	LIVER TONIFICATION	SQUAT JUMPS	FRONT KICKS	OBLIQUE V-UPS	SINGLE-LEG HIP RAISE
DAY 9	GATHER YANG	LUNGS TONIFICATION	DUMBBELL CURL SQUAT PRESS	ALTERNATING LATERAL LUNGE	GOLF SQUAT	SIDE LEG RAISE

PHASE 3 NIGHT TIME EXERCISE CALENDAR

	EXERCISE I	EXERCISE I I	EXERCISE I I I	EXERCISE IV
NIGHT 1	GATHER YIN	TURTLE BREATHING	GONG SPLEEN	YU BLADDER
NIGHT 2	GATHER YIN	TURTLE BREATHING	GONG SPLEEN	YU BLADDER
NIGHT 3	GATHER YIN	TURTLE BREATHING	GONG SPLEEN	YU BLADDER
NIGHT 4	GATHER YIN	TURTLE BREATHING	GONG SPLEEN	YU BLADDER
NIGHT 5	GATHER YIN	TURTLE BREATHING	GONG SPLEEN	YU BLADDER
NIGHT 6	GATHER YIN	TURTLE BREATHING	GONG SPLEEN	YU BLADDER
NIGHT 7	GATHER YIN	TURTLE BREATHING	GONG SPLEEN	YU BLADDER
NIGHT 8	GATHER YIN	TURTLE BREATHING	GONG SPLEEN	YU BLADDER
NIGHT 9	GATHER YIN	TURTLE BREATHING	GONG SPLEEN	YU BLADDER

CHAPTER 23

Buying Your Produce

Buying Your Produce

Before going into our eHealth Lifestyle Recipe section, there are a few critical points we would like you to embrace. Your awareness in selecting which produce ends up on your plate is essential and vital to your health and well being. Always check the numbered labels on your produce before purchasing to ensure that you're not buying potentially harmful foods. The first number in any sequence, on a label, determines how the produce was farmed:

- A four digit number beginning with **3** or **4** means the produce is conventionally grown, i.e., conventional use of fertilizers, pesticides and other cheap, deterrent chemicals.
- A five digit number beginning with **9** means the produce is organically grown, i.e., no use of chemicals or pesticides.
- A five digit number beginning with **8** means the produce is genetically modified. **LEAVE IT ALONE!!!**

Genetically modified foods (which we often refer as hybrid or heterotrophic foods) are riddled with yeasts and bacteria, which are the actual modifying agents that are, along with the new, invading DNA strand, inserted into the original cellular nuclear DNA, of the target produce, to transform it into the desired specie. When any food substance is altered at a molecular level, the effects on every other specie consuming it, is devastating. Cancer and all other cellular diseases are at an all time high, and there is no coincidence that their exponential increase is proportionate to the increase in consumption of genetically modified foods.

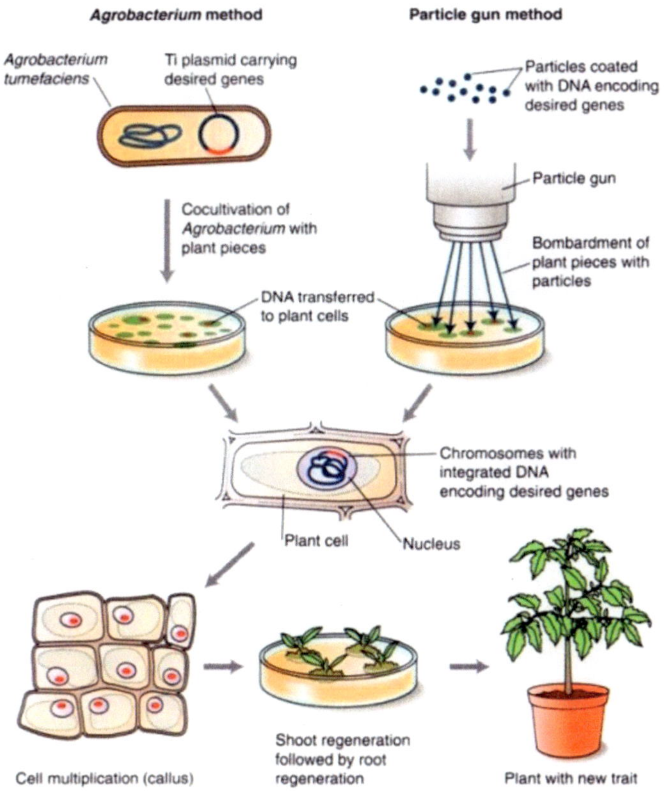
Agrobacterium method
Particle gun method
Agrobacterium tumefaciens
Ti plasmid carrying desired genes
Particles coated with DNA encoding desired genes
Particle gun
Cocultivation of Agrobacterium with plant pieces
Bombardment of plant pieces with particles
DNA transferred to plant cells
Chromosomes with integrated DNA encoding desired genes
Plant cell
Nucleus
Cell multiplication (callus)
Shoot regeneration followed by root regeneration
Plant with new trait

For More Information Visit:

www.electricphood.com

www.theelectricdocs.com

Made in United States
Troutdale, OR
11/11/2026

57125319R00090